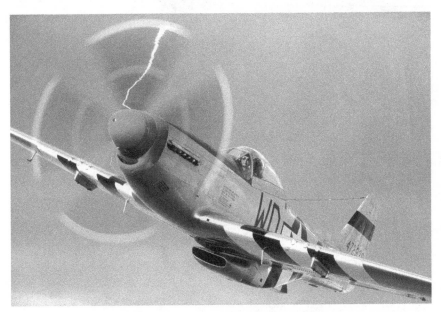

Lad on the cover of GHOSTS magazine. ©*PhilipMakanna/GHOSTS*
The P-51 was on the front cover of GHOSTS-1998.
Lad flying the P-51 photo near Dallas in September of 1996.

Lad Doctor's story should be required reading for every young man struggling with what it means to be strong, to be a leader, to be a man. Every stereotype of "manliness" can be found in Lad Doctor's youth and in each step of his career. His heroic accomplishments are straight out of a Hollywood script. Yet, when unimaginable tragedy tested him, he emerged even more heroic, physically limited but spiritually freed and empowered, a Godly man. There is no way of knowing how many lives Lad Doctor has forever touched and changed, but this book will certainly add to that number. I know it added me.

—*Office of Congressman Rob Woodall (GA-07)*

I know myself well enough when asked to which proverbial group I belong, talkers or listeners, I hit the listeners group—bullseye. Point being, I'm a really good listener. Listeners not only know when someone is "stringing some yarn," but they also record when something has already been said. I've known Lad Doctor personally for ten years—not once has he repeated a story. Not once. That makes Lad an amazing storyteller, but it also means he has the material from which to tell those stories. "Lad, what was it like to fly the P-51, or the P-47 or the Me 109 Messerschmitt?" "Lad, how did you get into the Air Race arena?" "Lad, the Vigilante had to be tough to bring aboard the boat." Any one of those topics, let alone a slew of others … well, they're a listener's delight.

One of the things I love about aviation is its breadth of field. Stretch the idea a little and you can get from general aviation homebuilts to the edges of space: stall speed of 50 knots to speeds I find difficult to comprehend. In creating this notion we have to associate people with events. Some were capable of X, some only got to Y. To my way of measuring, there were none more elite than the subject of this book—Lad Doctor. Youth of intrigue, Vietnam era Naval Aviator (in the Vigilante!), southern California banker, real estate developer, Reno Air Race Instructor & Check-Airman, Flight museum Chief Pilot. Cuss out loud, he even suffered his fate with poise, and class, and style. Remote Control airplane pilot, firearms master and small-town Texas building committee member.

I didn't even scratch the surface.

If you're only an arm-chair fan of the amazing field of aviation—and its respective icons—this masterpiece by Stella is a must read. Anyone within the field, set up a chair airshow style, sit a spell, and simply enjoy. You're about to read a great story.

Greg Storm
American Airlines First Officer
Commander, US Navy (ret)

I really did not know how much Lad really did accomplish, especially after his accident. I can tell you that I really thought that he was one of the most honest people that I ever met.

I do not really like to fly, but when he would fly me to Paso Robles for meetings, I, for some reason, was extremely comfortable with the way he would make me feel since I did not like flying.

The book really opened up my eyes on how many people he touched and on how many people wanted his expertise on airplanes.

Once again you did a great job in explaining all he accomplished and the book will be a huge success.

Frank Arciero, Jr.
Arciero & Sons, Inc.

I flew with Laddie many times. He is a dear and genuine friend. He was also a great pilot.

Phil Makanna
GHOSTS

I'm most proud of my father's strength and perseverance. There have been many memorable trips and outings with my dad over the years. Some that come to mind easily are: Indianapolis 500, skiing in Mammoth, Paris for a long weekend, Reno Air Races, lots of airshows and aerobatic competitions. We got scuba certified together. I helped him in the garage when he worked on projects, often handing him tools. I went to work with him when I was little and have many memories of hanging out at the racquetball club, playing backgammon or visiting construction sites with him.

–*Katherine Leah Doctor (Katie)*

Also by Stella Brooks

Unbelievable
The Unmasking of Dr. Harrison Miller Moseley

GROUNDED

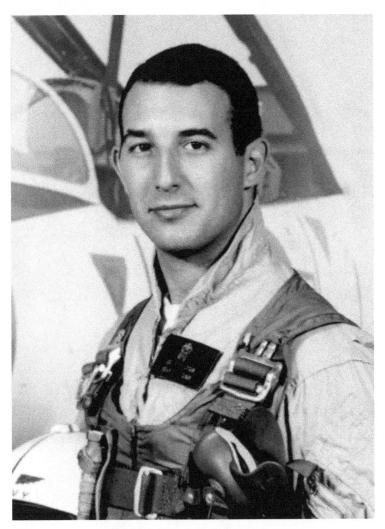

Laird Ashley Doctor, "Doc"

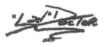

Now, I can see that all of those things were *by* the
Grace of God. Opportunities I thought I was
choosing to do weren't really my doing.

GROUNDED

A true story of a man who made the decision to live.

"God knew that the only way that he was going to get me to understand that I can't do it without Him was to prove it."

Stella Brooks

ISBN: 978-0-9996484-9-0 (hardback)
         978-0-578-77282-0 (paperback)
         978-0-578-77283-7 (ebook)

To mom,

Sarah Jean Florence Bennett.

She was the greatest, God fearing Christian

I have ever known.

She gave selflessly to others. Her children and
grandchildren were her priority and joy.

Acknowledgments

Lad's story covers a wide variety of subject matter, and because of this, many subject matter experts, as well as Lad's family and friends, have helped get his story told. To all of you, thank you for giving Lad the opportunity to inspire and move millions with his story of redemption and faith that could be theirs too.

Greg Storm, thank you for having the keen wisdom to see an awe-inspiring man and trusting me to bring your friend's story to the world.

Ben Merritt, you were the nucleus that brought everyone together. Without you, Lad's inspirational story might not have been told. Thank you.

Katie Doctor, and Lucas and Rylan Troup, thank you for sharing your father and grandfather with us. He is an inspiration and a joy to be around.

Leslie Schlom, Lad's cousin, thank you for sharing your Midget Racecar pictures. They give a visual glimpse into Lad's childhood.

Jim Miller (AHRF.com), thank you for sharing pictures donated to you by Leslie Schlom for your treasure trove of Midget Racecar pictures.

Phil Makanna, source of the amazingly beautiful pictures of Lad flying high. Thank you for sharing. They beautifully capture Lad's love and energy for aviation.

Frank Arciero Jr., thank you for sharing your memories.

April Feldman, California State University, Northridge. Thank you for providing much-needed documentation from Lad's days in the Sports Laboratory.

Craig Yancey, your wealth of information and brave honesty regarding your firsthand recollection of what took place that frightful day at Oshkosh added unbelievably important details that were not known till now. Thank you.

John Larsen, thank you for sharing your remarkable stories of working with Lad to create an absolute wonder—an apparatus that would allow Lad to fly again.

Michael Jouett, to whom Lad credits for being alive today. Thank you.

Milo Ruch, who can't say too much about this man. Lad's former assistant and special friend, Milo was Lad's go-to guy. He repaired everything from his wheelchair to his RC Planes, which they both enjoyed and have rich memories.

Terry Otis, thank you for sharing memories that added a special sentiment of days gone by. To this day, Terry and Lad remain strong friends.

Rick Millham, thank you for being our eyes on that fateful day at Oshkosh and sharing the outpouring of prayers for Lad.

Darlene Swanson for a beautiful cover.

David Hughes, your first-hand experience in engineering, aerospace and writing was the perfect mix needed. As with *Unbelievable, The Unmasking of Dr. Harrison Miller Moseley*, your talent is a necessary element.

CONTENTS

PART II

PART I

PART 1

Chapter 1

It All Started When ...

According to eyewitness reports, the [southbound] Corsair hit the Bearcat, one of the two airplanes that had come to a stop on the edge of the runway.

On impact, the Corsair sheared the right wing off of the Bearcat, which tipped up at a 45 degree angle before coming to rest facing the opposite direction. "The Corsair spun off to the [east] side of the runway and began cartwheeling into the grass, where it lay burning until emergency crews arrived," said John Lawson, of Louisville, Ky., who witnessed the crash.

"Two of them had stopped for whatever reason, I don't know why. The Corsairs were taking off and one of them just plowed right into the Bearcat," Lawson said. "I can't understand why they (the Corsairs) were cleared with a cross wind when there are two planes on the

runway."[1]

As Rose Yetta Shure hastily knocked on the door of Irene and David's small apartment, others followed closely on her heels. Their hands clutched her shoulders as they bobbed and weaved in an attempt to get a glimpse inside the small apartment before pressing through the door.

"Where is he?" Rose asked. She was an elderly woman and the family matron.

In the winter of 1942, in Cleveland, Ohio, Laird Ashley Doctor was the object of affection. As Rose Yetta Shure lifted her precious grandson into her arms for the first time, she could never have imagined what lay ahead for her sweet grandson, whom she loved so dearly. Inside the small apartment stood a large, close-knit Jewish family who were there for one reason: to see their newest member.

Laird Ashley Doctor was born on November 3, 1942. His life would be full of many twists and turns and hair-raising experiences. Decades from now, this baby would one day be protected by a new friend who would rock the foundation on which he was raised.

Wall-to-wall family had spilled into Irene and David Doctor's tiny apartment, many of whom were so successful that the Doctor's apartment on First Avenue could have easily fit inside any one of their houses. No one seemed to notice the cramped quarters because it did not matter; what mattered was family.

Laughter, cheer, and congratulations shook the windows as the family took turns coddling the baby. First grandma Rose, then cousin Iris, Morris Schlom, Rachel Schlom, Leslie Schlom, Max Schlom, Morris Shure, Charles Doctor, Harold Shure, and others.

Their apartment had the bare necessities and no more; that is how Lad's father, David Doctor, wanted it. He would live a life of honor, never taking a free dime from anyone. Irene and David would relocate from one apartment to another throughout their lives. Kitchen chairs were brought into the living area to accommodate their large family.

In the corner of the living room sat a significant piece of furniture, the radio. From it they enjoyed modern tunes and became updated on world events. Next to the radio stood a boy quietly taking in all the commotion and celebration.

The roar of conversation from anxious family bubbling with eagerness to see the newest member was heightened by Irving Berlin's latest hit, White Christmas floating through the air. It was quickly becoming as popular as his hit, God Bless America.

The family passed Lad around as if he were an antique vase. Rose impetuously lifted him from the arms of the last to hold him and began to calmly rock back and forth to the lively tunes of Glenn Miller, Jimmy Dorsey and other big bands dancing from the radio.

"Lloyd, come over here," Rose commanded, gesturing to the boy standing silently next to the radio. Lloyd was 11 years old, and his mother, Rose Shure, looked more like his grandmother than his mother. As she held her grandson, her youngest son pressed into her shoulder, his attention fixed on the baby in her arms.

"Meet Laddie," Rose said to her son.

A huge smile erupted on Lloyd's face.

"Hello Lairdie," he replied.

Even though everyone in the family called him Laddie, from that day forward, he would be Lairdie to Lloyd. This young boy had no idea how important he would one day become to Laddie.

Interrupting the happy-go-lucky tunes, a reporter's voice rose above the chatter.

"We interrupt this program for a special message."

The mood of everyone in the room suddenly shifted from high energy to somber. There was only one thing that could have pulled Rose Shure's attention away from her grandson, and this was it. She continued calmly rocking with the gentle tap of her toes against the floor, but her face told a different story while she listened to the emergency announcement. Everyone in the room stopped cold as they were drawn toward the radio.

Rose studied that piece of furniture as if she were looking at the newscaster square in the eyes.

"Gasoline rationing begins immediately," the newscaster announced.

Men combed their fingers through their hair, glancing at each other then back to the radio. "And under the command of Alexander Patch, the United States soldiers and Marines are finding it difficult to fight the Imperial Japanese forces in the dense jungles and tropical environment on Guadalcanal."

Almost one year ago, on December 7, 1941, the Imperial Japanese Navy Air Service had attacked the United States naval base at Pearl Harbor, killing 2,403 men. Rose's son, Norman Shure, was there. She had already lost one daughter from a ruptured appendix and a son to scarlet fever. The thought of losing another child was agonizing. She looked down at her precious grandson and prayed that he would never experience the horrific tribulation of war. What she didn't know was that Laird Ashley Doctor's life would be many-faceted. He would experience events others dreamed of, and people from around the globe would be drawn to him.

The room grew silent except for the voice of the radio announcer. Morris Schlom leaned forward in his chair with his elbows resting on his knees, his hands clasped together, chin resting on his hands with a stern gaze. Harold stood close by, leaning against the wall, hands in his pants pockets as he stared at the floor. Everyone in the room was deeply engrossed with the reporter's news.

Everyone except David. As he leaned forward in his chair to get a glimpse of his son, he became lost in his own thoughts. Though he lacked a high school education, David would teach his son everything he knew, including integrity and hard work, which sometimes meant working two or more jobs late into the night.

On July 2, 1935, he had dropped out of high school and enlisted in the United States Navy. The Depression was in full swing. As David slogged past the soup lines, he knew he needed a dependable employer, namely Uncle Sam.

Sometime later, while on leave from duty aboard the U. S. Submarine S-42 stationed in Panama, David had stopped by to visit his Aunt Ray. At that same time, Miss Irene Mildred Shure had dropped in to see her uncle, Morris Schlom. David's aunt, Rachel Cohen, and Irene's uncle were husband and wife.

After returning to Panama, David wrote Irene regularly and included pictures in an effort to include her in his world.

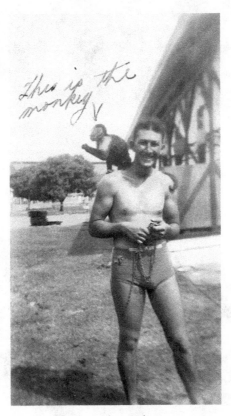

This is the monkey.
Compliments of Laird Ashley Doctor

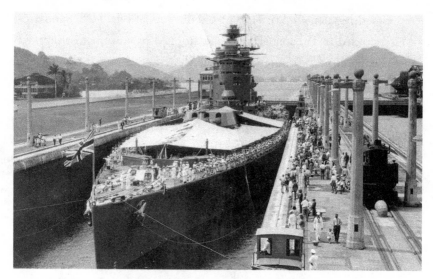

A British Battleship in the Panama Canal locks.
Compliments of Laird Ashley Doctor

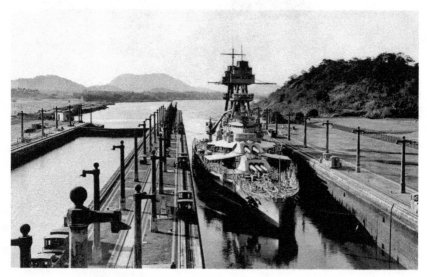

An American Battleship in the Panama Canal locks.
Compliments of Laird Ashley Doctor

For entertainment, while stationed in Panama, David played semi-professional baseball on the Isthmus League. He easily fielded a thousand and batted over 300, and somehow, from across the world, the Red Sox got wind of this 5 foot 7 ½ inches tall, left-handed first baseman. This sailor stood to gain a lot.

In 1939, the Boston Red Sox salaries ranged from $4,000 a year up to the two top-earning players: Jimmie Foxx, who earned $27,500, and Joe Cronin, who pulled in $27,000.[2] David was blessed with natural athletic talent that would excel him in every sport he played.

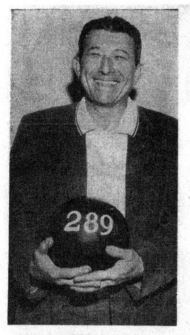

David Doctor rolled a 289 at Pan-Pacific.
It was the highest game in the 16 year history of the loop.
Compliments of Laird Doctor

DAVID DOCTOR, Wilshire with a spare, ten strikes and a nine count, rolled a 289, the highest game bowled by a Ben B'rith in Southern California thus far this season. Doctor carries a 150 average.

"My father had a chance to go to the major leagues," remembered Lad. "But life has its twists and turns."

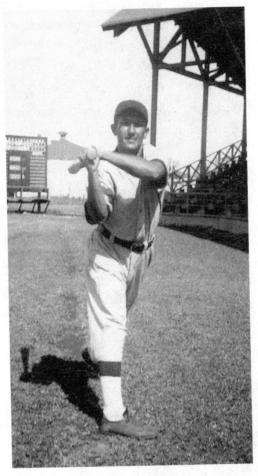

David Doctor, Panama.
Compliments of Laird Doctor

On May 26, 1939, using his travel allowance of five cents per mile, David Doctor was on his way home to Atlanta, Georgia.

Mr. and Mrs. Morris Shure, 1623 Eddington road, Cleveland Heights, announce the engagement of their daughter, Irene Mildred, to David Doctor, son of Mr. and Mrs. Charles Doctor, 3689 E. 154th street. The Doctors formerly lived in Atlanta, Georgia.

§

Suddenly, "God Bless America" began to play, abruptly shaking distraught moods and memories of bygone days and waking David from his memories of yesteryear.

The next day, David had just been home long enough to eat supper and sit next to the radio when Irene drifted into the living room. The dishes were washed and the tranquillizing music dancing across the room lured her into a hypnotic state of calm.

As if someone had just poured cold water over her face, she was startled out of her serenity and jolted back to reality as the nightly news interrupted the program to address unthinkable war stories of suffering and death.

Everyone was impacted by the malicious war and there was little hope of it ever ending. It seemed to go on and on, sucking the life out of every American.

As the family celebrated Lad's birth, they probably could have never imagined that those being praised on the radio that day for their war efforts would one day cross paths with their son. Four decades later, Laird Ashley Doctor's life would bond closely with many of the Second World War heroes. He was just a baby when his mother and father listened to the announcer enlightening them of a brave 19-year-old Texas girl, Florene Miller, who had her whole life ahead of her, but instead volunteered for service in the Army Air Corps. With striking beauty, she could have chosen any of the numerous "safe" occupations, but Florene had been raised in the cockpit and knew she would add value to the war effort. She was one of only 28 women who qualified for the original Women's

Auxiliary Ferrying Squadron (WAFS), later known as the Women's Air Force Service Pilots (WASP).

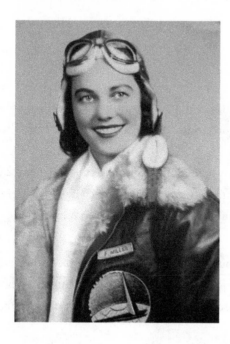

Florene Miller Watson.
Courtesy of Rebecca Wright.
Compliments of Laird Doctor

How could America ever grasp the sheer horror the troops were living? The evil they were fighting to keep it from America's doorsteps could never be understood second-hand. One day, Lad would understand, and he would have close bonds and intimate friendships with many who were talked about over the airwaves at this time.

Six months prior to Lad's birth, on May 4, 1942, Charlie Bond, a member of the American Volunteer Group (AVG), was fighting for his life. As fantastic as it would seem, Lad would one day call this Fighting Tiger a friend.

Charlie hopped in his cockpit, started his engine, and looked up to see a formation of 25 Japanese bombers heading right for the airfield. He sat there a moment, hand on the throttle, hesitating. His takeoff would put him on an intersecting path with dropping bombs.

"Hell, I can make it!" he said to himself. He rammed the throttle forward, racing to get in the air and away from the airfield before the bombs fell. In a maximum power climb, he finally got buckled into his parachute. He looked around. He was alone! None of the other Curtiss P-40 Tomahawk fighters had gotten in the air.

The bombers bypassed the airfield to drop their bombs on the city and made a long turn back to the south. There was no fighter escort to be seen, but Charlie picked up the second wave of bombers, another 25 in one big V formation at 18,000 feet. These were the ones he would go after.

Bond climbed 1,000 feet above them then dropped into a diving left turn toward the bomber at the end of the long right leg of the V. His first burst completely enveloped the bomber's fuselage but produced no fire, no smoke. Suddenly, the next two bombers in the V started streaming bluish white smoke, pretending to be wounded. The AVG pilots had been briefed about this trick, but this was the first time Bond had seen it. He ignored them and made another attack on his original target. On his third attack, the bomber's engine disintegrated into a flaming torch. The bomber slowed, fell out of line, and dropped into its final dive.

Charlie attacked the next bomber on the end of the V—and his guns quit. He had run out of ammunition. He made a 180-degree diving turn back to base feeling disappointed.

Suddenly, he heard loud explosions inside the P-40! He swiveled around. There they were! Three Japanese Zeros "firing like mad" from behind his plane. The explosions were their rounds piercing the fuselage fuel tank behind the cockpit and striking the armor plate behind his seat. The fuel tank exploded. Flames whipped through the back of the cockpit and up around Charlie's legs. He had to shut his eyes against the flames encircling him, but he got the canopy back, pulled the nose up, and rolled the P-40 over. The air stream pulled him out of the cockpit. He was tumbling when he pulled the ripcord.

He landed in a Chinese cemetery a mile and a half from the airfield….

The first Chinese to appear carried a big rock hidden behind his back. Charlie had to pantomime to convince the Chinese guy that he was friendly. The man led him to a nearby hut where the AVG's Doc Richards would later find him.

Bond made his mark on the AVG's history in his first weeks in Burma. At the local Baptist mission, he picked up a section of a British newspaper. On the front page was a picture of an Australian P-40, its lower nose around the air scoop painted brightly to resemble the wide open mouth of a snarling tiger shark.

Bond discussed painting the open mouth of a snarling tiger shark with his squadron mates and then with Chennault. The Old Man liked the idea and suggested the shark mouth be painted on all the AVG P-40s. In the end, Bond had to share credit for giving the tigers their teeth with 1st Squadron colleague Erik Shilling. At about the same time that Bond saw the photo, Shilling was looking at a magazine photo of another toothy airplane, this one a German Dornier bomber in the Western Desert. Shilling painted the teeth on his P-40 and showed it to Chennault. It was a case of great AVG minds thinking alike.

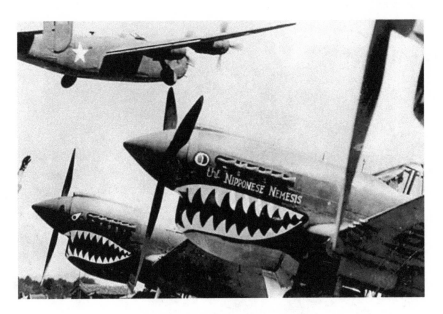

P-40 Warhawks, the staple of the
American Volunteer Group Flying Tigers.
Warfare History Network[3] Chapter 2

Chapter 2

Roots

It was number nine. Lad's grandmother's apartment was #9 on 2874 Mayfield Road and significantly close to the Doctor's apartment. Apartments were everywhere. There was little to no scenic beauty. Tall, plain buildings with little or no trees lined the street.

"Back then, families stayed together," remembered Lad. "My aunt lived down the street and a cousin directly across the street. They were everywhere and close by."

One day, while playing outside, a large hand reached down with force and grabbed Lad's small hand.

"My mother taught me, somewhat forcibly, that little kids do not get in the street," remembered Lad.

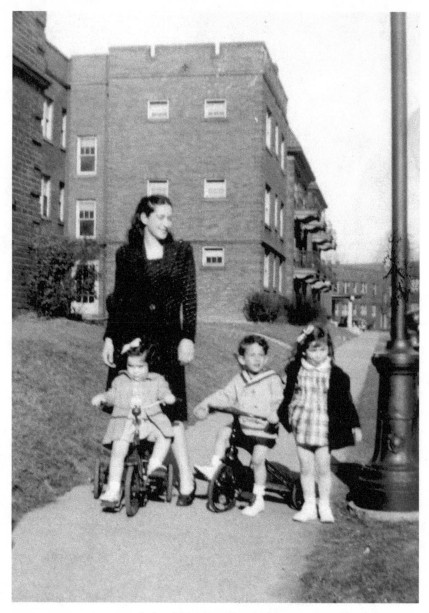

Lad and friends on First Avenue.
Courtesy of Laird Doctor

Back then, neighborhood roadways weren't as dangerous. It was a slower time. It was a one-car-per-household America. Fewer cars meant safer streets. Children were everywhere.

Sometime later, the Doctor's moved in with Grandma Rose and Lloyd. Lad's grandfather had passed away and Rose needed assurance that her youngest child, Lloyd, would have family close by if anything were to happen to her. The apartments were so close that it took longer to move the furniture up and down stairs than it did to drive the eight minutes to Rose Shure's apartment.

There was nothing special about it—two dark, red brick buildings with a flat roof, just like all the others. However, in the courtyard between the two complexes was a sidewalk forming a large circle from one building to the next.

Lad sat in the grass, clamped his metal skates onto the bottom of his shoes and clomped through the grass like Frankenstein, hoping the skates would not detach before reaching the sidewalk. He barely got rolling when Wham! He fell right on his face.

"I have poured a lot of cement," said Lad. "And it never cracks at the stress releaser."

Grandma Rose slept in the living room on a Murphy bed. It was a brilliant contraption invented by William Lawrence Murphy, a young man living in a one room apartment who desperately needed to be able to convert his bedroom into a room appropriate for any visitor. But, to be able to do so, the bed had to go.

By adding a pivot and counterbalance to his foldup bed, Murphy was able to hide it in the wall.

§

Finally, America had an opportunity to end the horrific war. On September 2, 1945, Lad was almost three years old when three young soldiers made a daring flight that could have cost them their lives. Colonel Paul Warfield Tibbets, the pilot, Theodore J. Van Kirk, the navigator and Thomas W. Ferebee, the bombardier, would bravely serve their country.

> *"At the age of 29, I had been entrusted with the successful delivery of the most frightful weapon ever devised," said Paul Tibbets. "One that had been developed at a cost of two billion dollars in a program that involved the nation's best scientific brains and the secret mobilization of its industrial capacity.*

> *"The scientists had warned that it would be unsafe to drop the bomb from an altitude of less than 30,000 feet. Because of the combined weight of the bomb and the fuel required for the 14-hour round-trip flight, the plane had to operate beyond its design specifications.*

> *"As the Enola Gay approached the Japanese city of Hiroshima, I fervently hoped for success in the first use of a nuclear type weapon. To me it meant putting an end to the fighting and the consequent loss of lives. In fact, I viewed my mission as one to save lives rather than to take them," said Paul W. Tibbets, Brig General USAF, Retired.*[4]

On September 2, 1945, World War II ended.

§

In 1947, five-year-old Laddie stole the show as the ring bearer for his cousin, Iris Shure and Bertram "Bart" Wolstein's wedding.

"Everyone admired Laddie," Iris remembered. "He took his job very seriously."

Little did she know her description of that small boy would define Lad throughout his life. Bart and Iris would go on to become extremely successful, creating a real estate empire, owning a sports team and performing philanthropy while based in Cleveland Ohio.

Later that year another celebration brought the family together.

"Yes," said Irene, when Lad asked her if he could taste the parsley dipped in salt water. "To celebrate the Jews' exodus from Egypt, you must also taste the Matzo, bitter herbs, charset, apple, roasted egg and lamb shank bone."

Lad obliged, then ran outside to play as the family celebrated.

"I clearly remember my mother preserving Friday night Sabbath candles," Lad explained. "It was always a lovely picture for me to see her alone at the dining table, washing the heat and candle smoke over her head while giving her prayers. Both of my parents were Jewish. In those days, there wasn't too much intermarriage going on."

Jewish festivals were celebrated and rooted in Lad's childhood.

"Look at it," whispered Lad.

"The Menorah was lit," Lloyd replied.

"Presents," Lad said softly.

Hanukkah was a time of celebration in the Doctor's home.

While Lloyd leaned over to gaze at the Menorah, he added, "A present every day for eight days."

"Nothing like the gifts given today," remembered Lad. "Small presents."

For a short period of time, Lad attended a small Hebrew school for a few hours a day.

Irene looked at the dreidel Lad had made at school and said, "That was a popular game when I was a child."

Long ago Jews were not allowed to worship God. But they found a way with the help of a top similar to the dreidel. As Jews secretly studied the Torah, they would throw the top and pretend they were playing a game to mislead the soldiers. The Hebrew word for dreidel is Sevivon, which means "to turn around," and the Hebrew letters on it mean "a great miracle occurred there." When the holy temple in Jerusalem was returned to the Jews, they could not find enough oil to keep the eternal light lit for a single day. But, miraculously, the insufficient oil lasted for eight days, giving them the amount of time needed to process more oil.

§

Because of his age, Lad felt Lloyd seemed more like a cousin than his uncle. Lloyd was fascinated with airplanes and worked well into the night meticulously building model aircraft.

"It was during the Second World War that people started thinking about flying," explained Lad. "Who flew before that? Few understood aviation in those days."

At a small table in the corner of the bedroom he shared with Lad, Lloyd quietly glued pieces of a model airplane together. Lad watched, deeply fascinated, as his "cousin" pieced together the model. There were many factors behind the force that pulled Lad out of bed that moment— the small boy with wavy brown hair and brown eyes crawled out from under the covers and onto his uncle's lap to watch. It was all new to Lad.

"Lairdie," said Lloyd. "Someday, I will fly a real plane."

Lloyd had introduced Lad to the world of aviation.

It was late and lights throughout the apartment complex were flickering off. But in the corner of the small bedroom the two boys refused to give up. Just a few more airplane pieces to fit together and it would be finished. Neither Lloyd nor Lad was in too much of a hurry to stop.

When Lloyd's father was alive, Lloyd had convinced him to take a ride to a deserted field so that he could tow a large homemade glider with the truck at a fast speed, then slam on the brakes. The speed, followed by the sudden stop, catapulted the large glider into the air.

From the rearview mirror his father was able to keep an eye on the plane as the truck sped down the field. Just as the dust began to cloud their view, the truck came to a screeching halt. Lloyd's nose was pressed against the back window so that he would not miss a moment of excitement…

BAM! The glider hit the back window of the truck.

§

Lad could not believe it. He dropped his schoolbooks on the table, his eyes fixed on a Stromberg-Carlson television. Grandma Rose had splurged and bought a television! It took patience slowly turning the knob until he hit one of the three channels. After he found the bandwidth, he turned the knob a tad bit more until he found the sharpest black-and-white picture he could get.

Rose, Lloyd, Irene, David and Lad watched The Milton Berle Show for the first time. At the time, no other technology, including indoor plumbing or the telephone, had spread so fast into so many homes.

The Howdy Doody Show was a huge hit. Lad enjoyed it almost as much as he idolized westerns. Howdy was a puppet adorned with forty-eight freckles, one for each state in the Union. "Kawabonga" was an expression invented for the show, and it surprised everyone when adults and children across the country began using this newly made-up word. But the most unforgettable moment was in the final seconds of the last show, when Clarabell, who, for years had communicated through pantomime and honking his horns, said, "Good-bye, kids."

§

"Irene!" Lloyd screamed.

She found her brother standing next to the Murphy Bed. Their mother had died in her sleep and her youngest child was horrified. Then Irene began screaming and crying hysterically. "Lloyd!" she yelled. "Take Laddie out of here. Hurry!"

"It was craziness," Lad remembered. "After that, and throughout my childhood, I had a real fear of dying in my sleep."

The Murphy bed would never be pulled from the wall again. It was no longer needed.

Lad was seven years old and thrust back into being an only child. Lloyd was now a young adult and had moved out. He quietly walked over to Lloyd's table in the corner, pulled the chair out and picked up where Lloyd left off. Lloyd's love of model airplanes had become important to Lad, too.

With no siblings and no one to play with, Lad's parents had given him permission to ride his bike while they were gone, as long as he stayed on the sidewalk.

He had never ridden on Middlehurst Road, and from where he stood, Middlehurst Road looked pretty inviting. As he admired his 1947 Roadmaster bike, he looked up and thought the small hill on Middlehurst Road would be a fun ride with plenty of sidewalk.

"Bicycles in those days looked more like motorcycles," remembered Lad. "The bar looked more like a fuel tank, slick fenders, a light on the front, a shelf on the back for books or groceries and a horn. It wasn't much of a horn."

He pushed the kickstand out from under the back wheel and carefully climbed on. At first, he was content riding behind the apartment, but quickly decided to turn onto Middlehurst Road. He started gaining speed until suddenly the hill did not seem so inviting anymore. He was fast approaching the busy intersection. It was getting closer and bigger and closer, but he froze at the wrong time and never thought to hit the brakes. He could see the Oldsmobile dealership on the right and a steel pole. Ahhhhhhhhh Whack! At full speed. Patrons from the gas station ran across the street and picked him up. Blood streamed down his throbbing chin. The tires left marks as Lad dragged his broken Roadmaster back up the hill.

After he arrived at home, he climbed up on the toilet so he could reach the small medicine cabinet.

"Laddie!

There he stood. His chin covered in gauze and tape.

Lad received four stitches.

Regardless of the stitches, the next morning he walked to school as usual. In the '40's, few families owned more than one car.

"Schools could not afford buses," remembered Lad. "In those days, it was a different America. It was a different world. Kids walked. You didn't have to be carted everywhere. And you never worried about being kidnapped or drive by shootings or someone selling you drugs. Those things were unheard of. I don't remember being in the house. We were told to go outside and play and be back before dark. I was painfully shy. I was not open at all, and I believe my feeling of loneliness stemmed from being an only child." He could sit in a classroom of 25 children and feel lonely.

From Charnock Elementary, he would pedal as fast as he could to the gun shop. After standing in front of the glass cabinet for some time, he would finally tear himself away, leaving behind his memory all over the glass gun case. Patrons could see the small hand and nose prints left behind by a small boy.

There was always plenty of entertainment during his walk home. There were carts topped with fruit and vegetables pushed along the road by local farmers. But it was the monkey that caught the children's attention. There he was, a man with a monkey sitting on top of an organ box held in place by a wide, thick, leather belt that hung from the man's shoulder. When the man turned the crank and the music began to play, the monkey would tip his small hat for coins.

When Lad arrived home, his father was ready to play ball.

Chapter 3

California Here We Come

Lad was about eight years old when the Doctor's moved from Ohio to an apartment on Glindon Road in Los Angeles, California.

"Better transportation was the key to the breaking down of the family unit," said Lad. "Families who once stayed together for a lifetime dispersed. You might call your uncle once in a while, or gather for a rare family gathering."

Mildred became a sales person at Bullock's Westwood Department Store, and David worked for Uncle Morris at Schlom-M.Schlom & Sons on West Jefferson Boulevard.

On the apartment lawn, David and Lad routinely practiced baseball. David was totally unaware that Lad did not enjoy the sport at all. But it was due to sheer fear. And the giant force behind that fear stood on one side of the lawn. On the other side of the lawn stood a small eight-year-old boy.

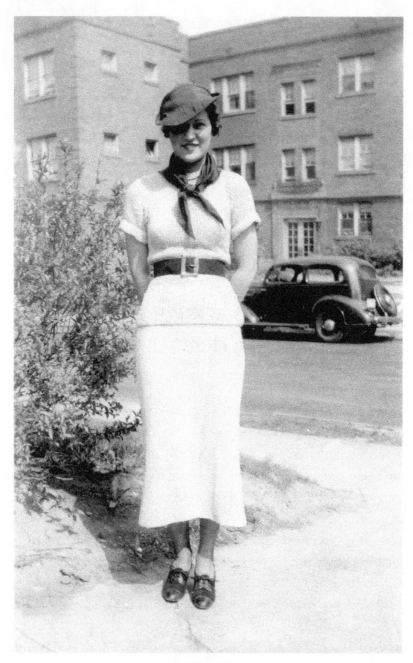

Irene Mildred Doctor.
Compliments of Laird Doctor

"When my dad threw the ball, you could hear the air grab onto the seams and manipulate it. Then, Whack! into your hand," Lad remembered. "And because of this, I was terrified of a baseball and did not want any part of it."

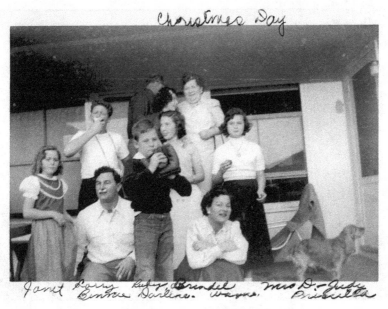

Lad with ball and glove.
Compliments of Laird Doctor

"I played any position the coach could put me where I was out-of-the-way. I played second base, once. The batter hit a ground ball that bounced, brushed against the top of my glove, then, BAM! Right in my face. When I came to, I looked up at my father."

"'Did I get him out?' I asked."

"'No, not hardly,' he replied."

Later, it was Lad's turn to bat.

"I do not like this at all," Lad muttered to himself.

Lad watched the pitch streak past his face.

"I just don't want that ball to hit me," he festered inside.

Ball one! The empire yelled.

STRIIIIKE!

Never moving to adjust his stance, he stood frozen.

"I do not like this. . .. I do not like this."

Ball two! Ball three!

The pitcher hid the ball in his glove, just under his eyes, staring at Lad.

"Don't hit me . . .. just don't hit me."

Ball four!

Lad stood frozen.

"Son, you have a walk," said the umpire as he pried Lad's hands off the bat.

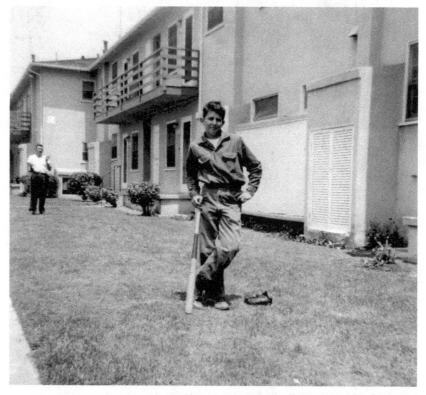

Lad and David Doctor practicing in the backyard of Glendon Road Apartments.
Compliments of Laird Doctor

The following evening, Jeff and Beau Bridges showed up to play with the group of children who gathered regularly on the lawn of Lad's apartment. As it turns out, though David and Irene lived modestly, they were surrounded by those who had the means to live lavishly. And that included family. David's work ethic did not go unnoticed and several well-off relatives offered him employment.

§

That evening, dirt flew all over everything and everyone, kicking up a dark cloud that irritated the spectators' eyes and hampered their view. But still they came.

David and Lad had arrived at the track long before the 18,000 customers were allowed through the gate. Lad knew the routine and the familiar sound of tires crunching across the ground as the teams rolled their midget race cars to the track. David and Lad were at the tracks so often that Lad could not remember a time in his life that he and his father were not there.

When the gates opened and the crowd spilled in, Lad knew that unforgettable and dangerous excitement was fast approaching. It was extremely rare for a child to be allowed that close to the action.

"The pit was no place to fool around," said Lad.

But Lad was allowed in the pit with a front row, up-close-and-personal view. He watched his father meticulously attach one end of a tow rope to the front of a midget race car and the other end of that rope to a tiny Crosley, a truck that had become popular during World War II because of gasoline rationing.

The midget race cars looked like the Champ Cars used in the American Championship Car racing circuit, which was associated with the Indianapolis 500, sporting a tight cowl that left no room for extras.

Lad watched as several Crosley's began towing their race cars. He studied his father as he carefully hung onto the back of the small truck pulling the midget car around the quarter mile track. The trucks towed the cars around the course a couple of times as part of the starting process; midget race cars did not have engine starters and had to be "pop started."

"There were no real organized crash crews," said Lad. "In the event of an accident anyone in the pit area would assist in extricating a driver from the car."

Lad heard the car start with a bang. He watched the driver edge up closer to the back of the truck to loosen the tow rope so that David, who was hanging onto the back of the Crosley, could bend down and unhook the rope from the car's front axle. Once the rope was free, David waved at the driver, who then slowed down so David could pull up the dragging rope.

Lad watched the race cars get into formation one-by-one.

Bam!

Off flew the cars at the sound of the starting pistol, and so did the dirt.

The first car had an advantage because those behind him found it difficult to see through the dust cloud as it pelted their faces. Sitting so close to the ground, the drivers felt every bump. David and Lad were very familiar and comfortable with famous drivers such as Billy Vukovich, Sam Hanks, Alan Heath, Karl Young, and many others.

"I remember a picture of Karl Young holding the winning trophy with me sitting on his lap," recalled Lad.

The dirt track was inherently unstable, which increased the excitement as drivers negotiating the tight corners fishtailed and slid, oftentimes spinning out, and finding themselves facing the wrong direction.

Lad cheered with the enamored fans as the cars struggled around the track, blasting dirt into the stands and onto the other drivers. Part of the excitement was watching the drivers shake their heads to free their eyes from the dust cloud in front of them. The sport was extremely hazardous because their head and neck were dangerously exposed above the car without the protection of a roll bar or a seatbelt, and deadly injuries happened often. Drivers were frequently thrown from their car or would run into a wall.

David always seemed to be employed by family, and that is what brought David and Lad to the track in the first place. Uncle Max owned Rose Midget Tire Company. His company manufactured the small tires the midget cars needed. Both owners and drivers sought after Max's knowledge and expertise. It was at Max's brother Morris Schlom's home where Irene and David had first met.

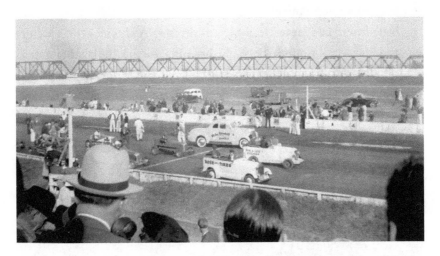

Rose Tire truck at a midget race at Southern Speedway in 1940, later known as Southern Ascot Speedway. The track was located near Atlantic and Tweedy Boulevard in South Gate and was torn down in 1942.

Compliments of Leslie Schlom and Jim Miller

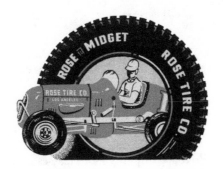

Rose Tire Company Logo.
Nostalgic Racing Decals, www.nostalgicracingdecals.com

Lad's cousin, Leslie Schlom, would occasionally hang out in the pit with Lad, but, surprisingly, Leslie's father, Uncle Max, rarely attended any of the races.

"Accidents were quite commonplace in those days," Lad recalled. "The worst accident I can remember was when Eddie Hadad went end-over-end more than once and didn't survive. There would be plenty of action in the accident department."

David and Lad never really left the races. At home, The Doctor's enjoyed hovering around the radio listening to the Indianapolis races, since they knew many of the drivers personally. Bill Vukovich was known simply as Billy in their circle.

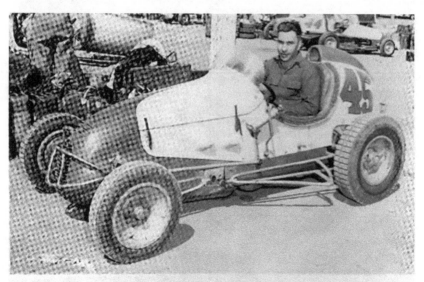

The original Bill Vukovich was called "The Mad Russian" but he was neither mad nor was he Russian. He's pictured at Milwaukee in a midget in 1950. (Bob Sheldon)

Bill Vukovich, "The Mad Russian."
The Vukovich Family Legacy[5]

"In those days, drivers competed in all classes of top-level racing and on all types of tracks," said Lad. "I think in many cases the month of May was the only time the drivers stayed in one place for any length of time.

It was more common than not to see many of the 500-mile competitors competing in the dirt race."

As a young boy, Lad understood the behind-the-scenes work that took place to produce a race and bring it to life for the millions of fans. He walked beside and watched the mechanics, owners and drivers working hard to bring it together. Watching them work beside his father brought the business down to his level. He grew up seeing the human side of the famous racers. Lad was more comfortable around famous drivers than he was with children his own age.

William Vukovich, Sr. won the 1953 and 1954 Indianapolis 500, plus two more American Automobile Association National Championship races. Several drivers of his generation referred to Vukovich as the greatest ever encountered in American motorsport.

Sam Hanks won the 1957 Indianapolis 500. He was a barnstormer, and raced midget and Championship cars. Hanks is believed to be the only Indianapolis 500 driver to race before World War II, serve in the war effort, then return to race again after the war.

Chapter 4

Following in Lloyd's Footsteps

On June 24, 1950, The United Nations Security Council unanimously condemned the North Korean invasion of South Korea. The United Nations came to South Korea's aid, with the U.S. providing 88% of the UN's military personnel.

The Korean War was the first in which jet aircraft played the central role in air combat. The P-80 Shooting Star, F9F Panther, Gloster Meteor and other faster jets replaced the World War II, piston-engine, propeller-driven fighters such as the P-51 Mustang, F4U Corsair, and Hawker Sea Fury.

Lloyd had received his wings back in 1948 and would go on to fly the XP-80.

Like a star athlete waiting to burst into the game at the last minute and shake everything up, the XP-80 burst across the sky out of nowhere and proved victorious.

In complete secrecy, the XP-80 was designed and built, complete with armament, in only 143 days. The successful secrecy of its development would be the start of the Lockheed "Skunk Works" program.

"Lloyd seldom spoke of his participation in the war," remembered Lad.

§

For ten cents, Lad enjoyed a double feature, cartoons, the news, and serials such as Buck Rogers and The Three Musketeers.

"I was always enamored with westerns," Lad said. "I immersed myself into the character. I felt I was the character, which is probably what got me interested in guns. I wanted a .22 rifle in the worst way."

"Boy, I wish I had that gun," Lad told his father.

"Absolutely not," David replied.

"July 27, 1953. I can remember the end of the Korean War," remembered Lad. "Because people stopped their cars in the middle of the street and started screaming." Lloyd returned home unscathed. But, since Lloyd was fascinated with planes, so was Lad.

But that wasn't all that Lad was interested in. He rode his bicycle to his cousin Leslie's house as often as he could to help him build his race car. Leslie Schlom was building a hotrod, and eleven-year-old Lad was right in the middle of it. Since both grew up at the tracks and both were captivated by race cars, Leslie needed the help of someone who knew what he was doing, and he knew his younger cousin would be a big help.

"Why don't you race?" Lad asked Leslie one day.

"My dad made me promise never to drive," Leslie replied.

§

"I was probably in my early teens when my uncle Eddie gave me my first gun," remembered Lad. "A German Luger 9 mm caliber. I shot the gun several times and can attest to the fact that it was not the most reliable shooting handgun in existence. You could not get through a full magazine of bullets without at least one problem."

It was during this time that Lad asked the family to call him Doc instead of Laddie. Everyone obliged, except for Lloyd, who would continue calling him Lairdie.

Lad was just a boy when tensions between the Vietnamese and the Japanese heightened to dangerous levels. Vietnam was the farthest thing from his mind, though. High school was a lonely place, and he would make it through without ever having a close friend. That was painful.

In 1957 Lad attended Venice Senior High School, the same school as Beau Bridges, the boy Lad had played with in elementary school. But Lad's shyness was so debilitating, that neither probably recognized the other.

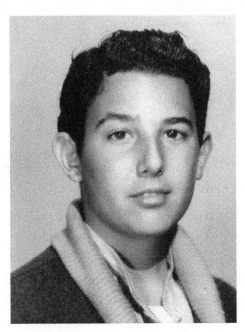

Laird (Doc) Ashley Doctor, 10th grade.
Compliments of Laird Doctor

If any of the boys at Venice High School had known that Lad sat in the pit at the midget races and knew Alan Heath, Sam Hanks and Bill Vukovich, the boys would have been lined up at his desk. He would have been that boy. The closest most boys got to the midget races was watching Mickey Rooney in The Big Wheel or Abbott and Costello in Midget Car Maniacs at the picture show. But no one knew, and having a friend his own age mattered.

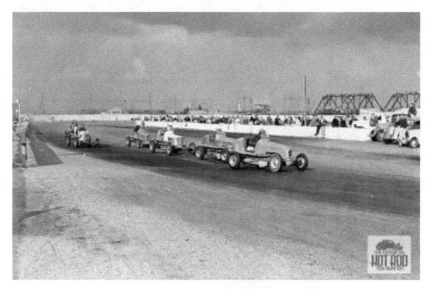

Cars raced turning to the left.
Compliments of Leslie Schlom.

"I never fit in. It was just a period of time," remembered Lad.
Lad hitched rides to school with total strangers.

"People picked up people in those days," Lad said. "There was never a thought in my mind that something could happen to me."

Lad had a natural talent for the life science class and it would be the only class he enjoyed. But he was so hung up trying to follow in Lloyd's footsteps that he missed out on his own talents. He built model airplanes, and now that Lloyd had become a successful NASA engineer, Lad had convinced himself that he too should become an engineer.

An award of $150 was shared by Elliott D. Katzen, Technical Assistant to the Ames Director of Astronautics, with Raymond K. Burns and Lloyd I. Shure of Lewis Research Center, for their invention of "A Protected Isotope Heat Source". The inventors were concerned with designing a protective container which would protect a radioactive isotope capsule from destruction during atmospheric re-entry, yet would allow the capsule to transmit heat to a utilization source in a space vehicle. This is accom-
(Continued on Page 2)

Lloyd I. Shure cited for his contribution to the invention, "A Protected Isotope Heat Source."
The Astrogram, January 6, 1972[6]

Turning a 1939 car into a hotrod was wildly popular. Lad did not have a driver's license, but he owned a hotrod. It was a beautiful 1939 Ford with a 1944 front end that his parents bought for him. The hotrod cost $90, and that was a lot of money for his parents to come up with, but David and Irene did without a few necessities to pull enough money together so their son could have a car. Lad loved it. The hood spanned half the length of the car, and the huge fenders swept over the top of the tires and almost touched the ground under the front doors. As Lad sat in class, he could not wait to get home, throw his books down, find his keys, run to the back of the apartment complex, and "fire that car up."

The neighbors had no need to hang out of their windows to know if Lad was home from school—they could hear him. Every day at 4 PM, Lad's Ford screeched up and down the alley, over and over.

One day, as he flew down the alley, an awful sound rang in the air. The grinding and squealing of parts was painful to the ears. Then silence.

Deafening silence. The car he loved was kaput. Lad had blown the engine before he could drive the car on the street. But since he had been around cars his entire life, he knew that car still held value. He used his ingenuity and know-how and began "parting it out." He knew the gauges were valuable, and by the time he finished selling parts, he had made $105.00. He sold the parts for more than his parents had paid for the car.

"If I needed anything," he reflected. "My parents would do without so that I could have it." It was a lesson Lad would not realize until later in life.

§

"Yes sir. I am very familiar with race cars," said Lad.

He fit right in. Stuart, of Stuart Dane's Race Cars, was intrigued with this young kid's mechanical know-how. The shop was on Venice Boulevard, just around the corner from school, making the job all the better.

Stuart Dane's garage was wide open, with two or three car bays.

"Air-conditioning, what was that?" remembered Lad. "If it was too hot you opened the door."

Lad assisted Stuart Dane in keeping privately-owned race cars in racing condition.

"His services were mostly limited to the drivetrain, engine, transmission, rear end, suspension systems, and brakes," explained Lad. "Stuart had an in-house racer he was trying to develop. It was a car he had designed to compete in a new racing class called Formula Junior. The project moved rather slowly and he never finished it. After I had left, I heard that Stuart was unfortunately killed in a bad crash at Riverside Raceway in Southern California."

Numerous Hollywood movies, television series and advertisements would be filmed at that racetrack.

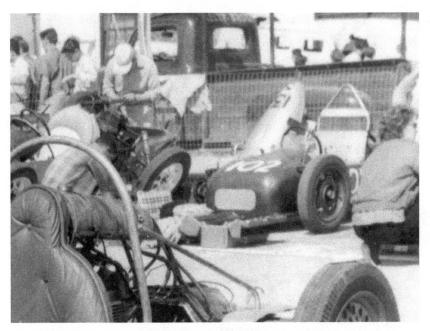

Stuart Dane's number 102 car, was driven by Mark Latker
at the Santa Barbara road races in March of 1956.
Compliments of Jim Miller

"I can see him!" said Lad.

On September 19, 1959, Lad and his father stood on the roof to get a better view of the freeway below. It had been blocked off for miles because the Soviet leader, Nikita Khrushchev, was visiting the United States and his caravan was approaching. It was history-in-the-making. They watched as the procession came into view until it had faded from sight.

Later, Khrushchev's motorcade pulled up to the studio.

The stars watched live coverage of his arrival on televisions that had been set up around the room, their knobs removed so nobody could change the channel to the Dodgers-Giants game. They saw Khrushchev emerge from a limo and shake hands with Spyros Skouras.[7]

For Khrushchev's entertainment, Frank Sinatra and Shirley MacLaine performed in a live performance of Can-Can. When the show ended, he observed that it was "exploitive and pornographic."

The room was packed with actors who clamored for a seat and a chance to dine in the same room as the Soviet leader. Elizabeth Taylor forgot her poise and manners and climbed on top of the table so she could get a glimpse of the famous visitor.

> *As the waiters delivered lunch....Charleston Heston, who'd once played Moses, attempted to make small talk with Mikhail Sholokhov, the Soviet novelist who would win the Nobel Prize in Literature in 1965.*
>
> *"I have read excerpts from your works," Heston said.*
>
> *"Thank you," Sholokhov replied. "When we get some of your films, I shall not fail to watch some excerpts from them."* [8]

§

The five-hour trip was worth it. His father didn't normally hunt, but David's friends had invited them to Mammoth Mountain for a little deer hunting. Mammoth Mountain had one of the longest ski seasons in North America and was frequented by many top ski enthusiasts as well as Olympians. It was a beautiful weekend just before snow season.

Lad had looked forward to the adventure so much that he got up early the next morning and started down the mountain. As he climbed down the side of it, he spied a good place to wait for a buck and made himself comfortable behind a fallen tree. Before he could get comfortable, he noticed deer tracks crossing the road just a few feet ahead. About that time a dozen or so does crossed the same path.

"They were so close that I could have knocked one out with a stone," Lad said.

However, does were not considered fair game and Lad knew that if a buck was amongst them, he would distance himself behind the herd. The buck never appeared, so Lad decided to follow the herd.

He stayed out of sight and followed them quietly as they meandered down the mountainside and onto a dirt road. After the herd crossed another road and started down the other side of the mountain, they suddenly picked up speed. Lad knew where he was and could have easily kept up, but it was getting late, so he decided to head back to camp. But the trip back up the mountain was very different than it was going down; the loose rocks were too slippery to get a foothold.

It was like trying to climb a steep sand dune, one step up, slide two steps back. After this little dance went on for a while, Lad was exhausted and decided his only plan of escape from that spot and return to camp would be to hike across to the dirt road and go all the way around the mountain.

"Sounded simple enough," said Lad. "But it was a lot farther around that mountain than it was to traverse down the side of it. Gravity helps going down and quite the reverse going up. I should've studied more diligently in the writings of Sir Isaac."

Lad was already exhausted when he decided to call it a day. He had hiked several more hours just trying to get back to the campsite before the sun completely disappeared. When he finally arrived, the men were seriously concerned and had been contemplating what to do.

"But no worries, and where was the bourbon!" Lad remembered.

§

There was absolutely no doubt in Lad's mind, after graduating, he would follow in Lloyd's footsteps and become an engineer. In May 1960, following the high school graduation ceremony, the seniors were required to meet in the auditorium to return their cap and gown and receive their final report card. The room was bustling with teachers, students and parents. As Mr. Bowers, Lad's Physics teacher, handed him his report card, he quickly pulled it back and said, "I will give you a passing grade as long as you promise never to be an engineer."

"I lied," said Lad. "I made that promise with no intention of keeping it."

His Uncle, Lloyd I. Shure, had done well as the Director of NASA Glen Research Center at Lewis Field in Cleveland, Ohio. He was also successful in publications and research, so Lad wanted to achieve the same. And his determination would smother the fact that he had a natural talent in science.

Even better, Lad could now drive on the streets of California.

Chapter 5

Sports Medicine

"I bought brand new books and they would sit on the back seat of the car," said Lad. It was 1960 at Santa Monica City College. "You know how when you open a brand-new book it cracks a little bit?" At the end of the semester, the student who would purchase his "used" books, would hear them crackle for the first time.

It would not take Lad long to realize that if he had studied in high school, he could have easily pursued an engineering degree. The college administration saw Lad's ambitions differently and advised that he take a year off to mature.

During this time, he continued his work for Stuart Dane and was a Summer Camp Counselor, which was a good fit for him since he enjoyed being outdoors. Work as a caregiver to a group of children would also play a pivotal role in overcoming his shyness.

The following year, Lad returned to school and once again pursued a degree in Engineering.

"Which was clearly not the direction for me to go," said Lad.

§

On January 20, 1961, John Fitzgerald Kennedy was inaugurated as the 35th United States President.

The youthful Kennedy administration is inexperienced in matters regarding Southeast Asia. Kennedy's Secretary of Defense, 44-year-old Robert McNamara, along with civilian planners recruited from the academic community, will play a crucial role in deciding White House strategy for Vietnam over the next several years. Under their leadership, the United States will wage a limited war to force a political settlement.

May 1961 - President Kennedy sends 400 American Green Beret "Special Advisors" to South Vietnam to train South Vietnamese soldiers in methods of "counter-insurgency" in the fight against Viet Cong guerrillas.

October 24, 1961 - ...President Kennedy sends a letter to President Diem and pledges "the United States is determined to help Vietnam preserve its independence..."

President Kennedy then sends additional military advisors along with American helicopter units to transport and direct South Vietnamese troops in battle, thus involving Americans in combat operations. Kennedy justifies the expanding U.S. military role as a means "...to prevent a Communist takeover of Vietnam which is in accordance with a policy our government has followed since 1954." The number of military advisors sent by Kennedy will eventually surpass 16,000.

December 1961 - Viet Cong guerrillas now control much of the countryside in South Vietnam and frequently ambush South Vietnamese troops. The cost to America of maintaining South Vietnam's sagging 200,000-man army and managing the overall conflict in Vietnam rises to a million dollars per day.

January 11, 1962 - During his State of the Union address, President Kennedy states, "Few generations in all of history have been granted the role of being the great defender of freedom in its maximum hour of danger. This is our good fortune..." [9]

As Lad laid out his best plans yet for a bright future, President Kennedy and others discussed getting rid of South Vietnam leaders, Diệm and Nhu, even though Kennedy knew South Vietnamese generals strongly disagreed and did not back an anti-Diệm coup.

January 15, 1962- President Kennedy had been asked if any Americans in Vietnam were engaged in the fighting. "No!" the President had responded without further comment. [10]

§

In 1963, Lad completed Junior College and transferred to California State University, Northridge.

"I don't remember why," said Lad. "But I changed my major to physical education, which led into Sports Medicine." With this career path, he would be living up to his name, and his world opened.

But, unbeknownst to millions of Americans, President Kennedy was secretly working an agenda that would forever impact the lives of millions of young American men, and Lad would be included. Dreams would be shattered and families destroyed because, even though U.S. advisors were fighting with South Vietnamese units, and U.S. pilots were flying combat missions in South Vietnam, President Kennedy continued to deny it.

Without Lad realizing it, his father's love of sports and exercise had now become a way of life for him. Lad's love for the outdoors and physical activity heavily influenced his decision to study physical education, which ultimately led him to Sports Medicine. Instead of reaching for someone else's goals, he began to pursue his own dreams and natural talents he didn't realize he had. He knew this was the right path, and for the first time in his life everything fell into place. He enjoyed what he was doing and he began planning his future.

Looking back, the one area of study that Lad had enjoyed in high school was biology and anatomy. And now he was enjoying both school and work. He was in his element. The required reading finally lost their crackle.

But, as Lad forged onward to a path of healing others, behind closed doors, President Kennedy sent signals to overthrow the Diệm government.

November 2, 1963, the president of South Vietnam, Ngô Đình Diệm along with his brother and advisor Ngô Đình Nhu were brutally murdered.

The tension between the Joint Chiefs of Staff and the Kennedy Administration worsened.

November 22, 1963, just twenty days after the assignation of Ngô Đình Diệm and Ngô Đình Nhu, John Fitzgerald Kenney was assassinated.

Lyndon B. Johnson was sworn in as the 36th United States President and would oversee massive escalation of the war while utilizing many of the same policy advisors who served Kennedy.[11]

During this time many households invested in fallout shelters while colleges stocked up with essential items such as food, water containers, first-aid materials and radiological equipment. According to an article in the Valley State Sundial, March 26, 1963, titled "Shelter Supplies Due within Ninety Days":

…Because the federal government dispenses only so much at a time in the way of supplies to each shelter area in the country, we will only have enough supplies to accommodate all the students for two or three days, he said.[12]

§

It was cutting edge, brand new. Dr. Holland, Dr. Rich and Dr. Wallace, professors at California State University, Northridge, asked Lad to assist in the design of a premier sports medicine laboratory. While working as their first lab technician, the doctors mentored Lad.

"Those were the early days in Sports Medicine," said Lad. "With grants and other forms of financial assistance we were able to dive into research immediately. Until then, there wasn't a Sports Medicine Department."

Finally, he realized his niche. He was driven to learn everything there was to know about Sports Medicine and the highly technical machines. He enjoyed helping others regain strength.

Lad was exactly where he wanted to be and had his career planned. Just as his mentors had suggested, he would complete his master's degree under Dr. Warvath, receive his Ph.D. under Dr. D.B. Dill at Nevada Southern, then return to California State as a professor in charge of the laboratory.

Lad could not think of a better career. The academic life offered the work he loved with the added bonus of having summers off.

During this time, sports medicine was cutting edge.

Page 12   Valley State Daily Sundial   Nov. 9, 1969

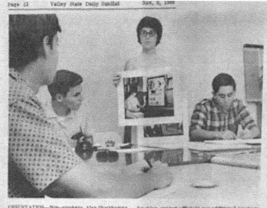

OBSERVATION—Non-smokers Alan Stockbauer, left, Tom Bosak and Charles Tarr are interviewed by Dennis Yavod before completing a written test on knowledge of smoking and health.

smoking project officials say additional smokers are needed for study, as many non-smoking students have signed up.

Students Puff, Then Huff as VSC Smoking Study Begins

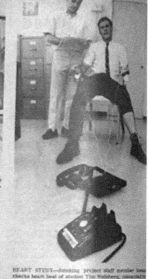

HEART STUDY—Smoking project staff member checks heart beat of student Tim Weisberg, connecting wire to Sherman Oaks research lab. Phoned signal goes to lab heart specialist, who compares smokers', non-smokers' beats.

spectrum

DAILY SUNDIAL

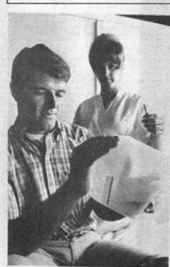

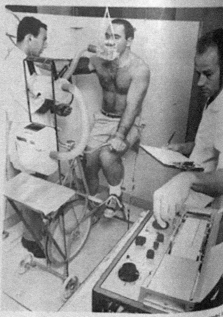

IN THE BAG—Student Allen Mitchell fills plastic bag with exhaled air. Technician Cheryl Barnes, rear, will later analyze contents to determine chemical differences in smokers, non-smokers breathes.

STATIONARY JOURNEY—Myron Miller exercises on bicycle ergometer apparatus while technician Laird Doctor monitors blood pressure and Dr. George Holland checks electrocardiogram.

Students who smoke are urgently needed for federally-financed program, say its officials. Volunteers will earn $10.

DAILY SUNDIAL PHOTOS

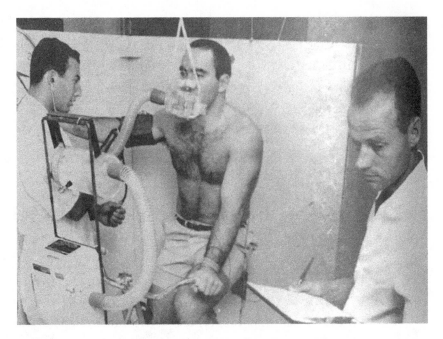

Laird Doctor, left, conducts a study on a willing college student facing him on a stool.
The newspaper caption reads: "Stationary Journey-Myron Miller exercises on a bicycle
ergometer apparatus while technician Laird Doctor monitors blood pressure and
Dr. George Holland checks electrocardiogram."

April Feldman, Archivist, University Archives, Oviatt Library, California State University, Northridge[13]

But the war efforts did not care if Lad had found his niche or not.
Dr. Holland, Dr. Rich and Dr. Wallace did care. Hoping that Lad could
stay and continue his work in the laboratory, they feverishly sent letters to
the Draft Board trying to convince them of Lad's value to sports medicine.
But while his mentors worked to keep him, Lad filled out the required
paperwork for the draft.

"Things were moving forward at a pretty good clip," said Lad. "I wanted
this career opportunity. Then, all of a sudden, I get this letter, 'Hey, we
want you' and I am expected to drop everything for the draft. The Draft
Board did not care—I was going to war. Case dismissed—good-bye. I had
90 days to report."

The entire situation was sad. The doctors' efforts failed. Lad was expected to leave the life he loved, forget his dreams and his family and go to war. On the surface, it would appear his future was totally out of his control, but what little control he had of his own life, he took charge of. Instead of relying on the Draft Board to place him in a position they felt best, he had a small window of opportunity to choose the branch of service he preferred.

Just as his uncle Lloyd had done, Lad went straight to the office of the Air Force. If he failed to get assigned to the service of his choice before the deadline, he would be placed where the military felt they needed him. He anxiously reported to the Draft Board in Westwood, California.

"We would love to have you," said the Air Force recruiter. "But we have a six-month waiting list."

"I only have 40 days," replied Lad. "I can't wait six months."

"Well, I tell you what," said the recruiter. "Why don't you go down to Alameda Naval Air Station near Long Beach. I hear that the Navy is always looking for cannon fodder."

"Those were his exact words, cannon fodder," Lad said.

The war got more appealing by the minute. Cannon fodder. His life was being pulled out from under him and he could expect to be treated as expendable in the face of enemy fire. David Doctor had taught his son a valuable lesson. If the curve ball hurts, pick it up and throw it back.

The next day, Lad was on the road making the 45-minute drive to Alameda, California, knowing that time was ticking. When he arrived, he found that the Air Force recruiter was correct, the Navy was sucking up as many potential pilots as they could and as fast as they could.

Once Lad received his notice and realized there was no chance of continuing with the ground-breaking study of sports medicine, he proactively enlisted in the Navy program, giving him the ability to choose the branch of service and role for which he would prefer. He took all opportunities to choose what little he could of his future. Before Lad could enter the program, he was required to pass the physical and fill out a lot of paperwork.

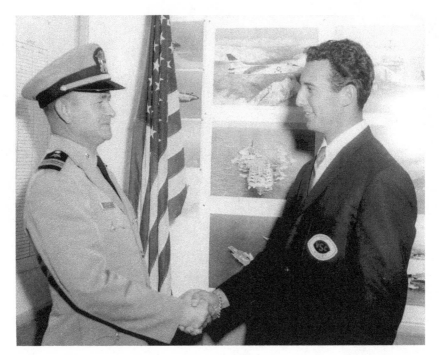

Inducted into the Navy.
Compliments of Laird Doctor

Chapter 6

Cannon Fodder

At least it would be a starting point. Since the Aviation Officer Candidate Program, "AOC," required a bachelor's degree, Lad reasoned with himself that when he returned to civilian life, he would be able to pick up where he left off in sports medicine.

In 1967, everything began to move quickly. Lad had received his diploma, transitioned from inactive to active duty and was expected to report to the Naval Air Station, Pensacola, in one week for the AOC program.

Despite their efforts, Dr. Holland, Dr. Rich and Dr. Wallace watched a promising young man walk away from two-and-a-half of the most promising years of his life. As Lad walked across the campus lawn, he stopped, turned toward the doctors, waved, and quietly marched off.

Lad made the most of the few days he had left before reporting for duty. In his 1964 Volkswagen Beetle, he left Santa Monica, California, and headed straight to Cleveland, Ohio, where family would welcome him with open arms. Then he jumped back in his car for a road trip to Atlanta, Georgia, to visit more family. He pulled through the gate at the Naval Air Station (NAS) in Pensacola, Florida, just seven days later. The moment his foot hit the pavement the yelling began.

During the next 18 months, there would be a lot of packing, moving and instruction. Irene probably knew from experience that her only child was being thrust into a war that could harm him in one way or another for the rest of his life.

"Going from civilian to military life is an experience," said Lad. "It's like stepping into an ice-cold shower. Your eyes get very large and very wide fast!"

"Sign here," said the Marine sergeant.

Lad began to sign his name when—

"Don't touch the line!" the Marine sergeant yelled.

Lad raised his hand away from the paper and began signing his name.

"I said, don't touch the line," the sergeant yelled.

"As I raised my hand higher and higher so that my hand would not rest on the line, my signature got worse and worse," remembered Lad.

"You're touching the line! You're touching the line! You're not supposed to touch the line! You scumbag, you're touching a line," he yelled.

"I finally realized that what the sergeant meant was for my signature not to touch the line, not my hand," Lad said.

"They bombard you with things you have to do. Drill instructors are screaming orders at you and you're just lost." Lad understood what they were trying to do. They were responsible for getting a group of young men trained and ready for war in a short period of time.

A civilian stood behind the chair with a razor in one hand and a pile of hair on the floor around his feet. It was Lad's turn. After his head was shaved, there was no need for a comb or a mirror. He looked just like the guy in front of him.

The first two weeks were referred to as Indoctrination. During

INDOC they learned commands, how to march, how to carry a rifle, how to handle a rifle, how to exercise, and more.

"Its purpose was to bring you into the military," remembered Lad. 90% of their physical training was conducted outside. "We lined up by height and marched everywhere; to breakfast, classes, events and just for practice."

The barracks were the same ones used during World War II. It was one of many that held five classes and several drill instructors.

Tommy Tompkins would be their drill instructor from the time they reported for indoctrination until they graduated as Ensigns.

"It was hot!" remembered Lad. "The screen doors allowed a breeze, if there was one."

"Eight minutes!" Tompkins yelled.

It was still dark. But, no time for stumbling around. They had eight minutes to get dressed and stand in formation outside on the grinder, which was a parking lot located directly behind the barracks used for calisthenics.

"Tompkins led us through calisthenics, running in place, jumping jacks, push-ups, sit ups, and some other kind of 'ups,' until we were good and tired," Lad said with a smile. "In the sand, we ran what felt like two to three miles. Far enough to get darn tired."

"We were often referred to as 'Scum Bags.' I am not sure whether that was proper or not, but a drill sergeant's vocabulary consisted of flowery short words that definitely got your attention. Whenever they called you, you answered! The name-calling and screaming were a little demeaning as we were college graduates." Lad enjoyed the entire experience. "Don't fight the system," he told others. "Just roll with it."

"You would have several guys at each sink looking over each other trying to shave quickly," remembered Lad. "It was quite a little picnic in there."

Time was not something Lad's class would ever have enough of. They had to get back to the barracks, empty the sand from their socks and shoes, shower, shave, make their bed, dress and fold clothes within a few minutes. T-shirts had to be folded in a perfect six-inch square. Then, back in the heat and on the grinder in their uniforms and in formation for inspection.

When the guys returned to their rooms, tired and dripping with sweat, they would find their clothes had been thrown in the middle of the floor.

Tommy had measured each shirt looking for the one shirt that was not quite a perfect six-inch square.

"No matter how careful you were," said Lad. "They were going to find something and your clothes would be in the middle of the floor when you returned. Here, remake this stuff... anyway. For two or three months we were run amuck. It was just as the recruiter had said, I was the 'cannon fodder' for the drill instructor. At one point, I was made the class leader."

§

POW! One powerful blast from an air gun was all it took. Lad and the other eleven members in his squadron had been marched up to a place called "NAMI," the Naval Aerospace Medical Institute. Naval Flight Surgeons were trained at NAMI, as well as Aviation Physiologists and Aviation Experimental Psychologists. NAMI was where experimental research took place.

Instead of receiving several vaccinations over time, the serums were all mixed into one powerful dose that took care of every shot needed. The recruits were given a shot. One single, powerful shot from an air gun into the arm.

When it was Lad's turn, the jet gun looked a bit more powerful than it seemed at the back of the line. Off to the side of the room sat an air compressor containing a gallon or two of liquid. A hose ran from the large container to the spray gun that would soon be pressed against their skin. The medical staff casually pressed the jet gun, which looked more like something a painter would use, against Lad's arm and pulled the trigger. *Pffff!* With a pulse of high-pressure air, a large dose of serum was blasted through the skin and into his upper arm muscles, leaving a deep bruise. It hurt terribly for days.

"It was very important that the physician place the nose of the gun against your humerus bone," remembered Lad. "It was shot under such high pressure that the liquid needed something solid to hit."

They missed the bone! As Lad and the other candidates waited in line before they could leave, they watched in horror as a candidate clenched in pain. The physician had not aimed the gun properly and the liquid came out the other side of his arm and splattered all over his chest. The pain was excruciating and the man had to stand there until the physician hit the right spot.

"I am telling you, my arm hurt. Ugh," Lad recalled. "Man-oh-man my arm hurt for a couple of days."

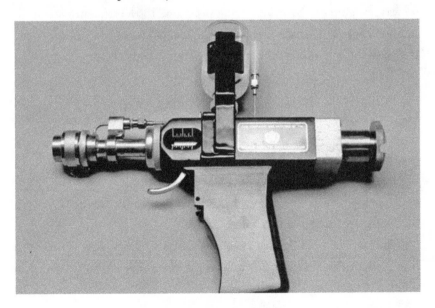

A 'jet gun' used during Vietnam.
The Orange County Register[14]

"Meals were one of the few aspects of life that wasn't dictated," said Lad. "You put your butt in any vacant chair. Chow was pretty good. Drill sergeants most definitely did not associate with students at meals or any other time. From our standpoint they were there to teach us military bearing, how to march, and generally make our lives as miserable as possible, and they were absolute experts at their job."

"Can you swim and at what level?" asked the Lieutenant.

Those who could not swim taught themselves very quickly. Only one guy in Lad's group had never swum. He was ordered to jump into water which was well over his head. He splashed and coughed his way back to the side of the pool, at which time the lieutenant ordered him to climb out.

"Jump back in the water," ordered the lieutenant.

"At this order the student was not quite sure if that was truly what was wanted or rather a little joke," remembered Lad. "It only took a nanosecond for the student to realize that if he didn't carry out the order he was not going to be in the flying program. To the student's credit, he jumped back in and, through the guidance of the instructor, he would later pass the one-mile swim test and swam like an Olympian."

§

"Wake up! Wake up!" yelled the nurse from an adjacent room.

Lad lay on his back at NAMI, alone in a dark room, his head resting on a block of wood. The temperature was a cool 65 degrees.

"Wake up!" she commanded again.

The staff at NAMI was measuring Lad's brain waves. Fifteen tiny pins—electrodes—were stuck to his scalp in various places, scanning his brain and recording information.

"Stay awake, Lad!" said the nurse.

"Why?" he asked.

"Because your brain patterns change when you sleep."

"I am in the heat all of the time," said Lad. "The cold feels so good, the lights are out, no one is beating me, no one is yelling at me. Oh, my goodness, this is wonderful. Can I stay here a day or two?"

"It is the same with all you guys," the nurse replied. "You are all so tired from the sun and running around with the sergeants hazing you all the time...."

"I was hoping she would shut up so I could go to sleep," Lad said, a smile crossing his face at the memory.

Then the electrodes were pulled off.

"NEXT!" called the nurse.

"And you are on to the next evolution," said Lad. "Staying awake was the toughest part of anything I had done thus far in the Navy."

The men would frequent NAMI. They were tested and measured for everything, including the length of their arms. Once NAMI could establish a norm, the data was used to help determine the size of a cockpit, astronaut selection and more.

"The good thing about NAMI was that it was air conditioned," said Lad. "And we got out of that damn Florida heat."

Chapter 7

Twelve Apostles

They made it through indoctrination. But there would be a hiccup.

"We called ourselves the Twelve Apostles," Lad remembered. "Because we had already been through the damn thing and now we had to go through it again."

Their class size of 12 didn't comply with the norm of about 20, so the military rolled them back into the next class and ordered them to repeat INDOC.

Once the Twelve Apostles completed INDOC a second time, they continued calisthenics and running, but classroom training would now consume most of their day.

"The 90-day training program was a great example of a perfect lesson plan to turn raw recruits into military officers in short order. Hence the term 90-day Wonders," said Lad. "In those days, our training had significant amounts of physical training as well as classroom instruction that covered everything from military etiquette to meteorology."

§

"So help me God." With those words, Lad was sworn in.

Three short months after his arrival at NAS Florida, Lad had become a Commissioned Ensign in the United States Navy.

The ceremony was complete with swords and big watches. In keeping with tradition, Lad, as well as the other officers, each paid their drill sergeant, Tommy Thompkins, one dollar for rendering their first salute as Designated Officers, Ensigns, or "Butter Bars" as they were sometimes referred to, because of the gold bar on their epaulettes that resembled a stick of butter.

The Officers were assigned to a Fixed Wing Training Squadron–1, or Squadron VT-1, and transferred to the Bachelor's Officer's Quarters (BOQ) at Saufley Field in Pensacola.

The first airplane Lad flew was the propeller-driven, single-engine, Beechcraft T-34, also referred to as the "Teeny-Weeny."

"There were no simulators for the Beechcraft T-34 Mentor in those days," said Lad.

It was imperative for the Navy to ensure that each officer was prepared for the next step. Therefore, each time new material was introduced, the officers were given a check flight. The result, or grade, consisted of either an UP or a DOWN. The Student Naval Aviators (SNA) needed an UP to move on. The grades were extremely significant because they would determine if the officer would be given a choice as to what aircraft he flew: Jets (JETS), Propeller Command (PROPS) or Helicopters (HELOS). After completing 17 flight hours in the T-34 Mentor, they would learn their options.

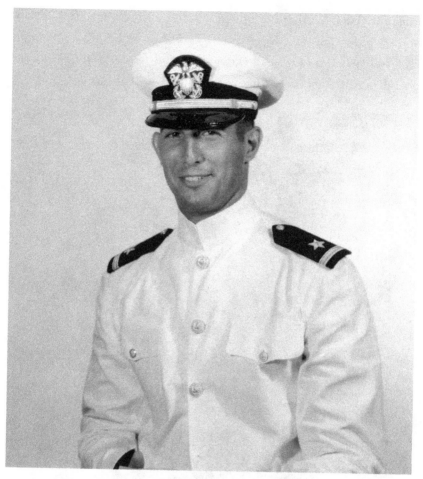

Ensign Laird Ashley Doctor, August 8, 1967.
Compliments of Laird Doctor

Lad was probably more like his father than he ever realized. Though he was thrust into an environment not completely of his choosing, he took his job seriously and excelled.

"Military life was easy for me," said Lad. "However, you don't drive the Navy, the Navy drives you."

It was a Friday afternoon. The Ensigns stood in line waiting for the phone to ring. They were told that there were 20 slots available at that time for JETS, another 20 for PROPS and 20 more for HELOS. The top 20 in the class were assigned to JETS unless the Ensign would rather fly PROPS or HELOS. Lad chose JETS and was soon on his way to Meridian Mississippi for Primary Jet Training, assigned to VT-7.

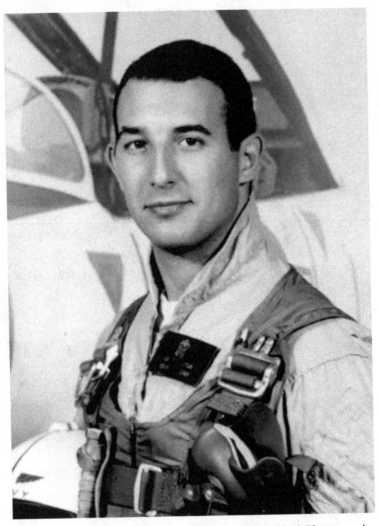

"I had not flown a lick when they took this picture," said Lad. The gear and helmet were not his and the plane behind him was nothing but a backdrop.

Compliments of Laird Doctor

They had the following weekend to pack, move to Meridian, Mississippi, and settle in the BOQ, but not until after the graduating class ahead of them had vacated the barracks.

"We had arrived in Meridian three days prior to check in," remembered Lad. "No one was around, so my best friend, Don, and I asked maintenance if we could take a few pictures standing next to the T-2A Buckeye in our new gear."

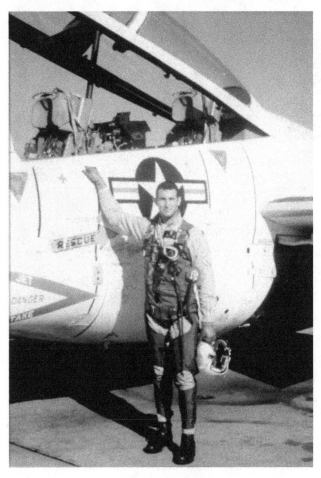

Newly-issued gear.
Compliments of Laird Doctor

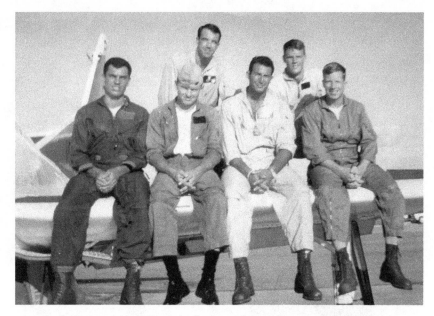

Lad's class on the last day in the first part of the jet program (T-2A Buckeye).
Lad, front row, third from the left. "I still have those boots."
Compliments of Laird Doctor

"In VT-7, we accumulated roughly 100 flight hours," remembered Lad. "The T-2A Buckeye was faster and larger than the Teeny-Weeny. It was a big jump from the T-34 to the T-2A."

The power in the jets was slowly increasing. Though the T-2A Buckeye was faster and larger than the T-34 Mentor, Lad would later learn that the T-2A Buckeye was still a relatively low-performance jet.

"However, it served its purpose," said Lad. "I learned the basic instrumentation and the feel of the plane."

The men were expected to process a lot of learning into a short period of time, and before they could get settled into one location, the Navy routinely uprooted them and sent them to another base. He studied every cockpit layout, the placement of every switch and gauge, and everything on the take-off checklist. Every flight was graded.

They packed their flight gear and moved a few steps down the hall to

VT-9 to master formation flying and aerobatics. From there, Lad returned to Saufley Field in Pensacola. Now assigned to VT-4, he mastered air-to-air-gunnery and worked on his carrier qualifications.

"To get to our classroom, we had to walk around the Blue Angel aircraft," remembered Lad. "And it would make our day to see a Blue Angel."

§

Neither had attended the University of California, Los Angeles, but both had friends there. Lad had the weekend off and while in Los Angeles accepted an invitation to an on-campus Greek party. While there, he met Dorothy Elaine Dahlgren.

"It was a big phone bill and a lot of letter writing," remembered Lad.

They had not dated or corresponded very long when Lad proposed.

On December, 1967, Dottie and Lad were married in a civil ceremony in his parents' apartment, just a few months after meeting.

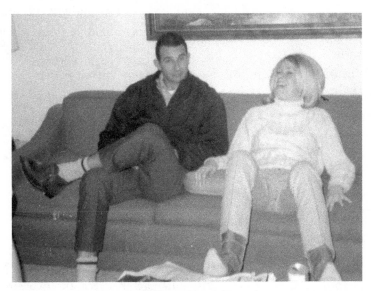

Lad and Dottie. December 1967.
Compliments of Laird Doctor

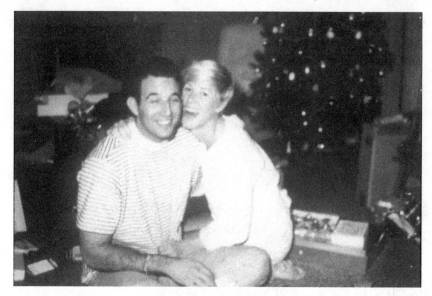

Lad and Dottie, Christmas 1968.
Compliments of Laird Doctor

"I asked for a week leave and they said, 'Are you kidding? You can have a *weekEND*,'" remembered Lad. Training was serious business and getting leave was virtually impossible. Dottie's parents realized that and were very welcoming.

When Mr. and Mrs. Laird Ashley Doctor arrived in Florida, Lad moved out of the Bachelor's Quarters and he and Dottie moved into an apartment.

§

Unlike the T-2A Buckeye, which had a single engine, the B variant had twin engines.

"The B's and C's were a much finer airplane in terms of power ratios and performance," said Lad. "The difference between the two aircraft was that the B variant had a Pratt and Whitney engine and the C had a General Electric engine. Early each morning, we participated in Field Carrier Landing Practice (FCLP) for hours and hours and hours flying the MOVLAS."

The mirror landing aid was a gyroscopically-controlled concave mirror on the port side of the flight deck. On either side of the mirror was a line of green colored "datum lights." A bright orange "source" light was shone into the mirror creating the "ball" (or "meatball" in later USN parlance) which could be seen by the aviator who was about to land. The position of the ball compared to the datum lights indicated the aircraft's position in relation to the desired glide path: if the ball was above the datum, the plane was high; below the datum, the plane was low; between the datum, the plane was on glide path. The gyro stabilization compensated for much of the movement of the flight deck due to the sea, giving a constant glide path. [15]

"At dawn, we ferried over to Bronson Field for Field Carrier Landing Practice," remembered Lad. "We were split into two groups with ten or less in each. Half of us flew in formation with an LSO to a training field and the other half and their LSO rode the bus, switching places upon return.

"As we drove through the gate, I could see a large number of fuselages and wings stacked in crates next to a small building, and the rest of the North American SNJs were inside a deserted building. Other than the student aviators, our Landing Signal Officers and a few mechanics, Bronson Field was a run-down ghost town. We were instructed to practice as many short approaches and touch and goes as a full tank of fuel allowed.

"Through the guidance of the LSO," Lad continued, "we flew the ball until we ran out of gas. It was intense flying. Touch and goes while flying the ball. The LSO was responsible for insuring we had what it took to go to the carrier.

"The LSO's were looking for a high level of proficiency and an understanding of his corrections while flying the MOVLAS. If I responded to their instructions without thinking, I would do just fine. If they wanted a little power, I gave them a little power. If they wanted a little right, I gave them a little right; little left, a little left; a little nose up, nose up. I did not have to think about it, just move the controls the amount they wanted. Once the LSO's were satisfied, I was ready to go to the ship.

"Our first carrier landings were on the *U.S.S. Essex* because the *U.S.S. Lexington* was out of commission. The *U.S.S. Essex* had the old hydraulic catapults," said Lad.

The flight deck was dangerously limited in length and hazardous for the pilot and all on deck. As one student landed on The U.S.S. Essex another took off.

"The LSO taught me (us) how to fly the landing mirror system via radio," said Lad. "Most, if not all, of the ships had been updated with steam catapults. Except for the old U.S.S. Essex. The difference being the steam catapult accelerates the airplane so that you had maximum speed at the end of the cat shot. The hydraulic cats started you out at takeoff speed and probably was losing speed as it went down the track. The difference was you got a real big jolt when the hydraulic cat hit the airplane. And in the steam cat it was a little softer as the power of the catapult built up running down the track. At any rate, though, it wasn't something we couldn't deal with. It was something we were told to look for. You were under the gun all the time. Our performance was always closely monitored. Any misstep could put you out of the program."

There wasn't much room for landing and taking off from the deck of a carrier. One careless misstep and a fighter jet engine could suck up a crew member or blast someone off the edge of the deck into the ocean.

"I remember absolutely nothing about my first carrier landing," said Lad. "I don't remember calling the ball or flying the airplane for that matter. I do remember turning downwind and final behind the ship and looking over the nose of the airplane and seeing another jet still in the landing area and a lot of commotion on the flight deck. I thought, 'Wow, look at what's going on down there.' Then suddenly, my airplane stopped. My memory of my first carrier landing was coming to a real quick stop."

Lad was now carrier qualified in the T-2B.

The Navy had two Advanced Jet Training Bases, one in Kingsville, Texas, and one in Beeville, Texas. Lad was transferred to Kingsville.

Chapter 8

Kingsville

Everything they owned was inside and on top of his Volkswagen Beetle. Dottie and Lad were on their way to Kingsville, Texas.

Lad arrived ready to fly the TF-9 Cougar assigned to the VT-21 Squadron for Advanced Jet Training. With strep throat. And to top it off, there was no base housing available. Their only option was to take a room in a dive motel until they were offered a trailer that a student ahead of him was vacating.

"It was a small, windy city with dust in everything and everywhere, including the inside of your car, your teeth and your ears," remembered Lad. Sometime later base housing became available, which was a lot nicer and situated close to the famous King Ranch."

§

"Under no circumstance can you take off with them in the airplane," answered the Commanding Officer.

"Don and I thought it would be pretty cool if we could take family and friends for a ride in a TF-9 Cougar," remembered Lad. "Of which we had little experience."

"However," the commanding officer continued. "If you promise to strap everyone in and brief them in case of an emergency, you can do an aborted takeoff."

"Wahoo!" Lad hooted. "We were just students so we didn't know a whole hell of a lot, but we thought we did. Putting on the equipment turned out to be a fun experience for Don's parents and wife, Dottie, her sister, and the wife of another student. It was a lot of explaining for a group who would never leave the ground."

Lad and Don took turns at the aborted take-offs. Each taxied to the end of the runway and accelerated at takeoff speed.

"We throttled back and taxied back," said Lad. "We did not stop to think that these were carrier airplanes. There were two issues happening that we had not thought of. The numerous dry runs on the hot pavement, the weight of the airplane relative to the size of the tires and continuous, hard braking and non-stop taxing was hard on those small tires. As I stood and watched Don, the next thing I knew, the TF-9 Cougar turns off the runway, rolls through the grass and stops."

Their hour of impressing ended with the crash crew coming to their rescue. A tire had blown.

The crew changed the tire and Lad and Don taxied home.

"We had not been in training very long when this incident took place. Or maybe we would have known better," Lad said, laughing.

In Texas, Lad dropped light blue, 25-pound practice bombs, fired rockets and aimed machine guns at a ground targets.

"All of my advanced training was in the TF-9 Cougar," said Lad. "The Navy depended on this aircraft during the Korean War. The TF-9 wasn't designed to be a trainer as the T-2 was. Modifications had to be made, including the addition of a second seat. I can remember getting in my first TF-9. The Cougar had the old analog gauges and green corrosion on a couple of switches."

The F-9 Panther was one of the first jets to land on a carrier. The difference being the Panther had straight wings and the Cougar had swept wings, a flying tail and an upgraded engine. Other than that, it was pretty much just like a Panther.

"It was a kick to fly," said Lad. "It had four 20-millimeter cannons in the nose and could carry a wide assortment of air-to-ground munitions. Flying the Cougar was a great experience and a rare opportunity because it was only available for that short period of time, in the Navy, anyway. We could feel the thumping of the cannons as they shot from the nose and smell the cordite as it filled the cockpit."

§

"In the TF-9 we did one touch and go and six traps on the U.S.S. Lexington," remembered Lad. "We called it the Grumman Iron Works. It was the only airplane I ever flew that I could have easily made an emergency landing in a forest without a concern. That airplane would have mowed those trees down. And that's why it was a Grumman Iron Works. In retrospect, it really was a fine airplane."

From NAS Kingsville, Lad returned to NAS Meridian, Mississippi, as a flight instructor in VT-7. As always he could not refrain from having a little fun. He once introduced a visiting student from the Naval Academy to Thermal Barrier and Hydraulics.

From the back seat of the T-2A, Lad asked the Ensign, "Do you know about the sound barrier?"

"Yes sir," answered the student.

"Are you familiar with the Thermal Barrier?" questioned Lad.

"No sir," the student replied.

"We are going to go through the Thermal Barrier," Lad warned, with tongue in cheek.

While the plane was pointing straight down at a high altitude, Lad turned on both the defroster and heater. As the airplane picked up speed, 180-degree air filled the cockpit.

"Can you feel the Thermal Barrier?" Lad asked.

"Yes sir. I can feel it!" replied the student.

"The old Thermal Barrier." Lad smiled.

"In the T2A, regardless of the airspeed when you turned off the hydraulic boost, holy moly, it was a handful," Lad said.

"Would you like to take over and fly the T-2A?" Lad asked the student.

"Yes sir! Could I really?"

Unbeknownst to the student, Lad turned off the hydraulic boost and there would be nothing the student could do to get the airplane to move.

"Sir, I don't understand what the problem is."

"Let me take control," Lad directed.

He quickly turned the hydraulic boost back on and whipped the airplane around.

"You need to hit the gym and work on that wrist and forearm because there is nothing wrong with this airplane," Lad told him.

Chapter 9

The Vigilante

From Mississippi, Lad transferred to NAS Albany, Georgia, for A-5 training. "The TA-4's were Tinker Toys compared to the A-5," Lad explained.

> *"The airplane was very complex and there was a lot to learn. It was by no stretch of the imagination a simple piece of machinery to fly. ...it just wasn't all automatic in that thing," remembered Lad.*

> *"It had tremendous capability for what it was designed to do and it did it very well."[16]*

The A5 Vigilante was one of the most beautiful aircraft to ever grace the skies. It was also the largest and fastest airplane to operate from an aircraft carrier, and it was the most complex aircraft the Navy operated.

"And this fact will still hold true when the Navy starts to receive its newest fifth-generation aircraft, the F-35," said Lad.

The original configuration was contracted to be a strategic nuclear bomber, and during that time the A5 hit a new world altitude record of 91,400 feet, surpassing the existing record by over 3 miles. The amount of knowledge the pilot and Naval Flight Officer would be required to obtain and retain required a long stint in ground school.

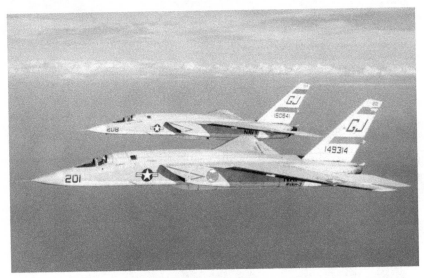

Lad and a friend flying the A-5 Vigilante, in formation.
Lad is flying the plane in the back.
Compliments of Laird Doctor

The Vigilante introduced more new and advanced designed features than any other aircraft in history: a specially designed fuselage configured for Mach 2.2+ flight; sharp-tipped, swept-back engine inlets for peak supersonic efficiency, with the first variable front and rear ramps to control the internal profile and throat area; a fully-retractable refueling probe in the forward fuselage; and major structures and frame components built out of titanium.

The Vigilante featured one-piece wing skins machined from aluminum-lithium alloy, and it used nitrogen instead of hydraulic fluid in some of the hottest parts of the airframe. A one-piece, bird-proof, Mach 2.2+ capable canopy was made of stretched acrylic, and the engine bays were gold-plated to reflect heat.

The Vigilante was controlled by the first production fly-by-wire flight control system, and it carried an airborne digital computer for bombing and navigation computations. This was the first Bomb-Navigation System with an inertial auto-navigation coupled to radar and television-sights for check point verification. It also featured the first operational heads-up display (HUD), the first fully integrated auto pilot/air data system and the first monopulse radar with terrain-avoidance features.

Performance

Speed: 1,320 mph

Service Ceiling: 52,100 feet

Crew: Two

Range: 2,050 miles

Wingspan: 53.2 feet

Height: 19.37 feet

Empty Weight: 37,489 pounds

Maximum Weight: 79,588 pounds

Power plant: Two J79-GE-10 turbojet engines

Thrust: 17,859 pounds thrust each

Later, major modifications were made to the A-3J/A-5A/A-5B to add sophisticated, electronic reconnaissance capability.

"The reconnaissance capability was contained in a fairing under the fuselage called the Canoe," said Lad. It contained a side-looking airborne radar, vertical, oblique and split-image cameras as well as active and passive Electronic Countermeasure equipment.

The inertial navigation system, combined with an automatic flight control system, enabled the RA-5C to fly precise courses, skimming along at tree-top level or zooming above 50,000 feet, where it could take damage assessment photos, each marked with the latitude and longitude of the plane at the time a picture was taken and later used as directional guidance to the photographed location.

In 1963 the RA-5C Vigilante began a new and dangerous mission of tactical reconnaissance to retrieve critical information required by the carrier task force. 23 Vigilantes went down. The RA-5C had the highest loss rate of any Navy aircraft during the Vietnam War. The hazardous pre-strike photography was dangerous, but the danger was offset by the element of surprise. Post-strike photography was even more dangerous because the Vietnamese gunners were ready and waiting. They knew when the smoke cleared the jets would return for vital bomb damage assessment, making them easy targets. But once the RA-5C's had returned to the ship, the electronic and photographic information was collected, processed by the electronic intelligence data handling center and analyzed by specialists.

Because of the high attrition rate, North American Aviation was paid to reopen the Columbus, Ohio assembly line for an additional 36 aircraft. Only 156 Vigilantes were ever constructed.

"We used to do what was called Ride the Landing Gear Handle," said Lad. "Our hand rested on the landing gear handle because the instant the airplane left the ground a few feet, we had to get the gear up immediately or exceed the gear door speed. It wasn't a landing gear limitation, it was a gear door limitation, because the gear door was run by a hydraulic jack. If I broke the jack, it could potentially cause a hydraulic failure. Following the gear coming up we had to raise the flap. The airflow alone could raise the flaps into their 220-knot limitation speed. Getting the flaps up before they were pushed up by airflow was difficult on your first takeoff.

"I'm lifting the flaps with the landing gear coming up and that thing going so damn fast," said Lad. "The whole take-off is so fast it's unbe-

lievable. You take off with an experienced RAN talking you through the takeoff because as I recall our first check was 100 knots before we got to the midfield arresting gear. [17]

"If I had failed to reach 100 knots before reaching that gear, I would have dropped the tail hook because the airplane wasn't accelerating properly," said Lad.

"On that first flight we went to full basic engine, releasing the brakes. As the aircraft started to role we put on full afterburners. And the reason is because the brakes would not hold the airplane while in full afterburner."

"If you didn't release the brakes, all you would do is start skidding down the runway. So the brakes must be released to start rolling and then engage the after burners. Or at least that was our procedure." [18]

Lad received cues from the RAN (Radar Attack Navigator) regarding the take-off procedures.

"Spool up the left engine," said the RAN.

"It's coming up," said Lad.

"Temperature roll back," he said.

"Got it," Lad responded.

"Pull your engine back," he continued.

"And you're going really fast through this stuff. And he is talking you through it. And you're trying to find the gauges, for crying out loud. Even though you had all this ground school, now you're in a real airplane and you're fumbling around a little bit. And I had an A-4 chasing me. The squadron used four TA-4's as chase planes. I released the brakes and shoved it into full afterburner and those things lit off."

In a Vigilante, the cockpit is located forward of the engine a significant distance. If the pilot's helmet fits tightly, instead of the tremendous noise from the afterburner, he hears a slight swoosh.

"During all of this, I'm looking for the nickel gauges," remembered Lad. "So that I would know the position of the turkey feathers. If they were not completely open during afterburner, the engine would melt. And you would have a big fire going on back there."

"100 knots, 100 knots," yelled the RAN.

"I looked over and was past 100 knots," remembered Lad

"ROTATE! ROTATE!" he commanded.

"I was still back at engine run and this guy is telling me to rotate," said Lad.

Lad experienced the powerful acceleration of the Vigilante.

"...it was a real hazy day below the clouds," remembered Lad. "There was a cloud deck 5-7,000 feet, something like that, and it was kind of broken to scattered. It wasn't a bad day at all. But my chase pilot, Lt. Commander Kulkie, said, 'When you pull up,' because the A5 is a lot faster than the A4. That's for darn sure," Lad said. "'When you pull up, just don't go through the clouds and level off,' the Commander said. I remember pulling back," said Lad. [19]

Lad had the gear coming up when he attempted to raise the flaps which were already up, which brought the droops up and—

"He had me level off and make a turn so that he could join up with me," said Lad.

On another flight, Lad was in the front seat flying the TA-4 while the instructor yelled demands from the back seat. Lad was chasing an A-5 Vigilante.

"I want to show you something about the Vigilante," said the instructor.

He radioed the pilot of the Vigilante, "Cruise at 350."

Lad kept up easily in the A-4.

Then, he told both pilots, "When you get to 3-2-1 power, go to full burner level flight."

"And we did that and the A-4 stayed with the Vigilante longer than I thought we would," remembered Lad. "Then, the Vigilante opened the gap."

Clearly the Vigilante was going to be faster than the A-4, the aircraft just didn't pull away immediately.

"You know, the TA-4 kept up pretty well," said Lad.

"Go to 450 knots level flight," the instructor continued.

"That A5 disappeared so damn fast it was unreal. I mean when he hit burner, he leaped ahead of us. That airplane was so far ahead of its time."

§

"We were staging out of NAS Norfolk, on the U.S.S. Kennedy, for carrier qualifications," remembered Lad.

"On my first catapult launch, the moment that I was catapulted, I was maneuvering the A-5 to full burner, shooting for an airspeed around 350 and 450, a two G pullup, and all of a sudden the Grimes light came out of the socket and landed on the right side of the console. I had a complete cockpit electrical failure. After I started to level off and turn downwind, I picked up that damn light and stuck it back where it went. I needed to call the ship, but now the radio didn't work.

"'Holy moly, now what's wrong with this damn airplane,'" I thought.

Lad knew and followed through every procedure needed in the case of an electrical failure. It helped that Lad knew they were in a VFR pattern (Visual Flight Rules) and that a plane was in front of him. However, he now had Bingo fuel and needed to land immediately. But that wasn't going to happen because, on the U.S.S. Kennedy, the airplane ahead of him had a hydraulic failure and was stuck in the wires.

"I got close enough to see that that aircraft was not getting out of the way," Lad explained. He knew that by the time the deck personnel cleared the disabled jet past the foul line it would be too late.

"The LSO was trying to communicate with me, but I was a 'nordo' (no radio)," said Lad. He was out of fuel, out of time and needed to somehow convey this to the LSO. Lad decided to descend and waggled his wings in an effort to alert the LSO.

"I was at Bingo Fuel (the amount of fuel available to reach a designated airfield suitable for the A-5, and nearest to the ship). When you reach that designated fuel state and you are not aboard the ship you immediately aborted to the designated Bingo Airfield. As the ship moves, the fuel needed to reach an airfield is constantly changing. In some cases, the designated airfield may also change. The Bingo Field we were using for that day was NAS Norfolk, Virginia. I went into after burner right across the flight deck and got just past the end of the ship accelerating to 350 to 450, I did a 2 g pullup that tagged the vertical speed indicator at the rate of 6000 feet per minute.

"The altimeter indicator was having a difficult time keeping up with the rate of climb. It would spin a couple of times. Then it would move slowly. Then it would stop and then it would spin a little bit. I was climbing to 23,000 feet as the optimum altitude, and that lagging altimeter would read around 10 and 13,000 feet.

"I pulled the engines back because the thing was climbing so damn fast. This allowed the altimeter to catch up. I rolled out at 23,000 feet. I was just amazed at how fast it went up like that. I mean the nose is up and all of a sudden, the power comes on and this thing just climbs and you go 'WOW.' The capability, power wise, was amazing.

"Upon landing the aircraft, the problems were easily fixed. Unfortunately, the ship was finished with flying for the day. I was told to return the following day with the next group that was going out for carrier qualifications," remembered Lad.

When used as a reconnaissance plane capable of speeds faster than Mach 2, Lad was flying a weaponless jet, forcing him to rely completely on his piloting skills and the aircraft's speed to get him out of harm's way.

Their motto was, *"Unarmed and Unafraid."*

Lad knew his stuff. He could discuss in intricate detail the aircraft's mechanics, how it handled and the secrets to flying such a powerful plane. He remembered what would happen at particular altitudes and at varying speeds and changing accelerations. He had an in-depth knowledge that would make him one of the elite pilots.

Chapter 10

Hey Doc You're a Father

"Hey Doc you're a father."

In 1971, Lad was stuck in Washington, D.C., when his daughter, Katherine Leah Doctor, was born at the Naval Air Station in Albany, Georgia.

Katie was two days old when he was able to see his little girl for the first time. Dottie and Katie were still in the hospital when he arrived.

"Military is rough on families," said Lad. "Too much time apart. I was gone for almost a year one time, followed by another year with a short visit home in between."

The Naval Air Station in Albany, Georgia, was the home of Commander of Reconnaissance Wing One (CRAW-1), the wing commanding all the RA-5C Vigilante squadrons. While there, Lad worked on his Landing Safety Officer (LSO) qualifications by grading and waving aircraft during Field Carrier Landing Practices.

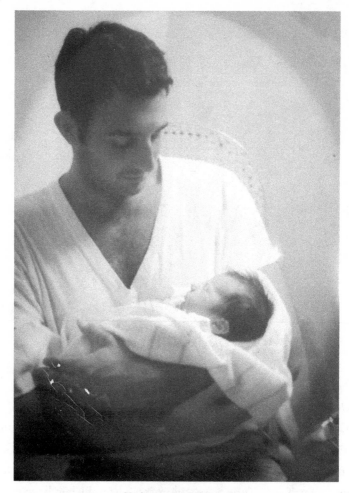

Katherine Leah Doctor
"Life changes abruptly at that point," Lad said.
Compliments of Laird Doctor

Lad and Dottie had been married four and a half years and Katie was just a little older than one month when he was deployed to Vietnam.

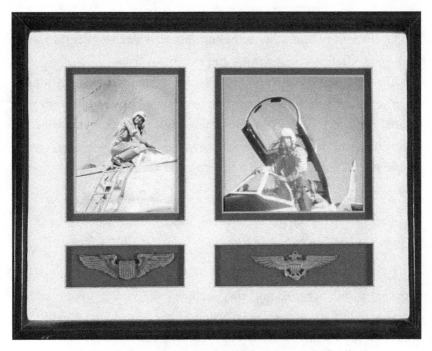

Lad created a similar photo with his wings to match Lloyd's.
Seen on Lloyd's photo is a note to Lad that addresses him as "Lairdie."
Compliments of Laird Doctor

Actress Jane Fonda would earn the nickname "Hanoi Jane" after she
made a trip to Vietnam to protest the war and was photographed sitting
on an anti-aircraft gun used to shoot down American pilots and planes.
Years later, she stated, "I am proud I went to Vietnam when I did. I am so
sorry that I was thoughtless enough to sit down on that gun at that time
and the message that it sends to the guys who were there and their families. It's just horrible for me to think of that." [20]

Because Vietnam was a political war, many American soldiers were treated
horribly upon their return. When in uniform, it was common for U.S.
civilians to yell hurtful remarks at the men.

"We had thousands of guys come back with missing limbs," said Lad.
"Talk about post stress. Nobody had heard about post stress, nor treated it,
even though all of those guys probably had it."

They deserved help. They had been in combat 24/7, cursed with jungle disease and humidity, never knowing who was for or against them, and Agent Orange would destroy and take many lives.

They did not volunteer to join the service, and after living through horrific suffering, instead of returning to an appreciative home, they were treated like the enemy. Their home, the people they thought they were giving up their life for, turned them away.

In Hurd Park, New Jersey, a small plaque reads,

They served, they fought, they died and received neither their country's glory nor their country's compassion. May this small plot of ground serve as a special tribute to them. Viet Nam Dec 1961 – Mar 1973

Lad received his share of grief. Shortly after returning home, he attended a military wedding that included the raising of the swords. Afterwards, Lad and a close friend, who was still decked out in his military uniform, stopped at a local bar. His friend had experienced more than his fair share of action in Vietnam and had been awarded many medals.

After his friend had a few drinks, a patron started harassing him for his involvement in the war. The patron hurled insult after insult. The next thing Lad knew, his Marine friend had drawn his sword and was chasing the heckler around the bar.

It was at this time Lad decided to drop the moniker, "Doc." But he left behind more than his nickname—he was done with flying. Not only did he lose all interest in flying, he didn't even go near an airport. Lad packed up his family and returned to southern California to pick up where he had left off in sports medicine.

Chapter 11

Done with Flying

He was done.

Because of the war, Lad had flown one of the highest-performance airplanes, and he had been on more than his share of aircraft carriers, too. He was grounded and planned to stay that way. Nine years earlier, Lad's world had been extremely different. He was back home now and eager to pick up where he had left off. He walked briskly across the lawn at California State and straight into the Science building.

"Science can move at a pretty fast pace," said Lad. "Dr. Holland and Dr. Rich thought time had passed me by. It really upset me." Lad had not joined the military on his own accord. It wasn't a stepping stone to further his career. It had taken him from ... everything. He eventually found a job handling large commercial loans for one of the major U.S. banks.

Around 1977, David Doctor had a friend who was a member of the Condor Squadron at the Van Nuys Airport and thought his son would enjoy becoming involved with this small group of mostly World War II fighter pilots. But Lad was done with flying. Period. He had a family and a job that took all his time and energy.

§

World War II had separated a group of guys who had grown up together, enlisted in the Air Force together and flew for the National Guard together. They reunited after the war and formed the Condor Squadron at the Van Nuys Airport in California.

Lad eventually conceded to his father's suggestion. When he saw the Squadron clubhouse for the first time, he could not believe how close it was to the runway. The clubhouse was painted a camouflage design and sand bags were piled around bombs that stood at attention beside the doorway.

"The building was phenomenal," said Lad. "It was grandfathered in so the airport could not get them out of there. I don't think the FAA liked them that close to the airway."

Every Condor member owned an AT-6 Texan and flew in one of two squadrons, one representing the American 31st Pursuit, with striped tails, and the other group portraying German fighters. The groups flew nose-to-tail behind the lead plane, performing the same loops and rolls and other aerobatic maneuvers while maintaining their positions. Besides formation flying, they also enjoyed fighting each other. Condor Jim Modes enjoyed perfecting the aerobatics.

"The paint schemes on the planes were at the discretion of the owner," Lad remembered. "It reflected a particular squadron or a famous pilot." The Condors believed that if you could fly an AT-6, you could fly any WWII era single engine airplane.

Lad was hooked.

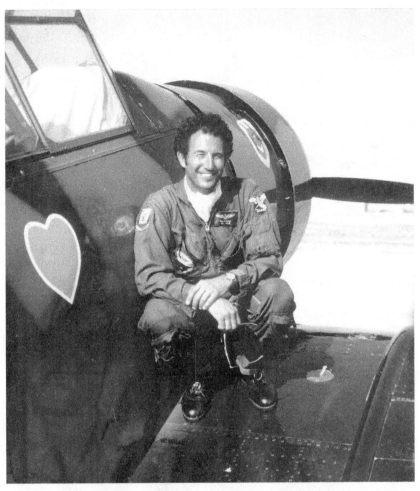

Founding Condor Dick Sykes' AT-6. The heart was
the work or design of the original German pilot.
Compliments of Laird Doctor

Every Wednesday he relaxed with the Condor Squadron in lawn chairs on the edge of the taxiway and watched airplanes land just a few feet away.

"I told them all about you," David had told his son.

"I don't need to be involved in anything flying," Lad had declared adamantly.

Now here he was, sitting with these World War II heroes, many of whom David and Irene had learned of three decades earlier from the radio standing in the corner of their apartment. The Condors performed at airshows and staged mock dog fights. As time went on, newer members lacked the necessary military pilot training.

Condor Charlie Beck raced at the Reno and Mojave Air Races, in the Unlimited Circuit. He and Jim Modes co-owned the Candy Man, a P-51 Mustang outfitted to race. The stars and stripes painted on the P-51D air racer Miss America were designed by Gene Clay in Honor of the U.S. Air Force Thunderbirds. Howie Keefe purchased the plane in 1969 for $25,000 and named her Miss America. He sold the P-51 in 1981 for $200,000. One announcement over the PA system at Reno was all it took to sell her.

"It's not just a Mustang, it's a P-51," said Greg Storm, Commander, U.S. Navy and Lad's good friend. "It's extremely rare. Very few get the opportunity to fly a P-51, but everyone who has flown would like to fly one. This is one of the greatest aircraft ever flown, ever built."

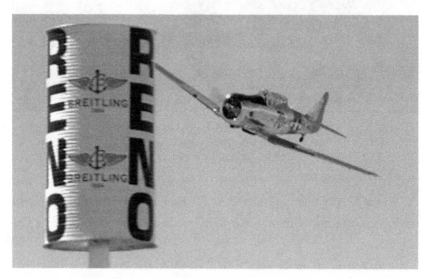

An AT-6 racing past the pylon at the Reno Air Races.
Compliments of Laird Doctor

Through the Condor Squadron, Lad served as the president of the T-6 Racing Association and as an FAA-designated check pilot for the Reno Air Races, and would do so for 18 years.

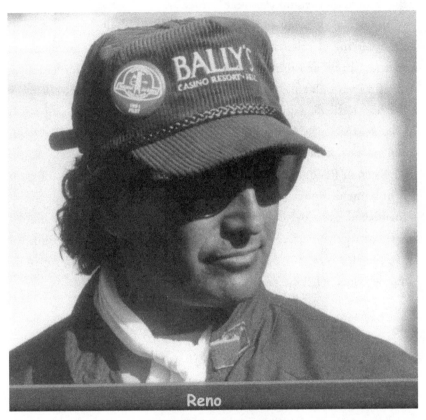

At Reno wearing a Corsair cap.
Compliments of Laird Doctor

"Every year, on September 15th, my body wakes up and needs to be in Reno," said Lad.

Charlie Beck became Lad's best friend in the Condor Squadron and allowed Lad to race his plane. Clay Lacy had a collection of planes used in numerous movies that can be spotted by his initials 'CL' on the tail.

Because Van Nuys Airport became extremely busy due to Los Angeles' population explosion, the Condors changed their departure strategy, shifting from formation takeoffs to taking off one at a time, creating a long string of aircraft. They flew north over the hills toward the high desert where they would chase each other.

"When you're flying in formation you are generally pretty close to each other and can therefore signal each other as to what is taking place," said Lad. "But when the aircraft are spread out and not in formation, it can tend to be a bit more hair-raising, dangerous if you wish, especially when the individual pilots come from various backgrounds and levels of flight experience. There can be hours of boredom interspersed with moments of sheer terror.

"When in Reno, I would frequently bump into a retired U.S.A.F pilot by the name of Robert 'Bob' Hoover, who was known to drink at times," remembered Lad. "Because of some weird ass shit he did, the FAA hoped he would receive medical attention and diagnosed as medically unfit to fly in the airshows. But instead, Bob went around the FAA. In Australia, Bob was issued a license and flew in the airshows anyway."

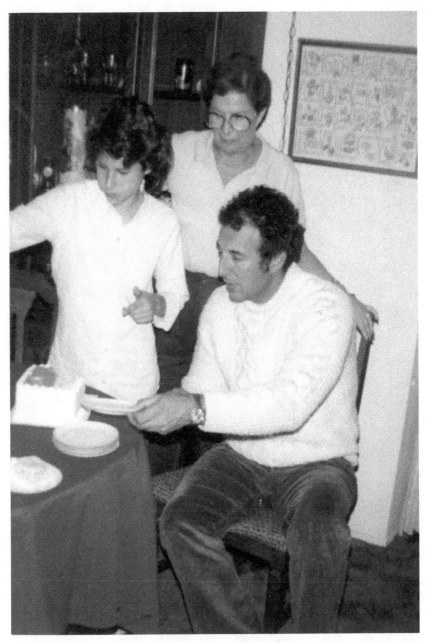

December 1983. Katie, Irene (mom) and Lad wearing his favorite watch.
Compliments of Laird Doctor

PART II

PART II

Chapter 12

Well, Maybe Not

"Passengers were not allowed on the race course," said Lad. But when the races were over, Lad sat in the backseat of Charlie Beck's P-51 while he warmed it up.

"The Reno Air Races came out of the Golden Age of Aviation as a means of determining the flying characteristics of new designs," explained Lad. "Lockheed, McDonnell Douglas, Pratt and Whitney, Wright Airplane Engines, and others used the Air Races as a proving ground when considering the purchase of an inventor's airplane designs. After World War II, private individuals took over air racing for the sport.

"Following World War II, hundreds of P-51's were parked in the desert to be used for ingots," Lad said. "The government practically gave them away for roughly $1,000.00. The customer got a P-51, the spare engine and 55 gallons of fuel. Fill her up and fly away."

§

Gary Meermans and Harold B. Loomis decided to start a T-6 racing association to help promote the T-6 class of racing.

"We called Hal the 'Skyatola,'" said Lad. "He ran T-6 Air Racing."

Gary Meermans, chief pilot for United Airlines, was the instructor and check pilot for the T-6 class. He was the only FAA check pilot for T-6 racing when it exploded in popularity. He knew Lad knew his stuff and would never cut corners, so he asked him for help.

"Whatever you decide is what I will do, pass or fail," said Meermans.

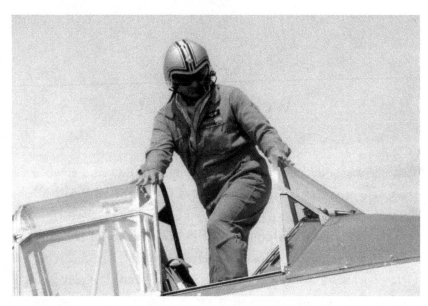

Lad flew in his first T-6 race in 1981, and Gary Meermans
raced the same plane the next year.
Compliments of Laird Doctor

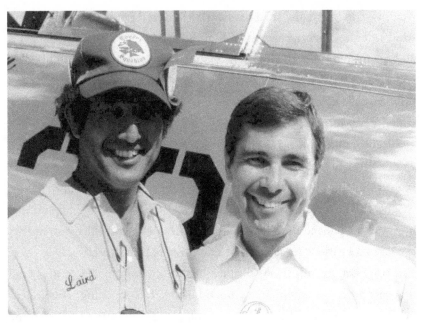

Lad Doctor and Gary Meermans.
Compliments of Laird Doctor

As time went by, Lad and Gary grew even more concerned for everyone's safety. In T-6 racing, pilots fly extremely close to each other. First time civilian pilots who had never flown in formation were now standing in line to race their new toys. So Lad and Gary developed a "must-have" baseline of skills every pilot had to pass before they were allowed to race. With the growing popularity of the sport, Gary feared that if an accident occurred at Reno while on his watch, it would jeopardize his position at United Airlines.

In 1982 Lad became president of the T-6 Racing Association, Inc. while maintaining his role as the check pilot and a respected source called upon by The Federal Aviation Administration Airshow Coordinator for technical input. Lad made certain these critical responsibilities were given the scrutiny needed for the next 18 years.

There were seven T-6's in each qualifying heat. They had more pilots wanting to race than they had room for, so Lad used a process of elimination to whittle down the numbers. Lad felt he had received affirmation in his ability and judgement from high-ranking pilots when they told him, "If you give a guy a check ride and pass him, we're comfortable racing with him." This level of complete acceptance meant so much to Lad that he would never forget it.

"I appreciated that. I would not let pilots who could not fly with a certain level of expertise enter the race," said Lad. He conducted pilot evaluations from the backseat until pilots began removing them to reduce weight. A volunteer pilot would serve as a leader so Lad could determine how well the pilot could stay with him, which was part of the requirements.

"We had various levels of pilot skill for sure," said Lad.

"Stop! Let me out," Lad yelled during one evaluation. "How many tail draggers have you flown? How much bullshit can you sling? If you can't taxi better than this, there is no way you can fly. You can't get me to the runway without doing a half a dozen ground loops. You would have killed everyone on takeoff."

With the elimination of the backseat, Lad had to lead the pilots through the process in a pace plane.

"Racing was demanding and dangerous in the T-6s," said Lad. "The planes were dangerously close when going around the turn, so I intentionally set up the race to keep from having accidents." The rigid rules Lad put in place created the safest environment possible. "A collision would have been a guarantee if I had allowed the pilots to ram around the pylon like a gaggle in a small airspace."

Like the Olympics, there were three award categories: silver, bronze, and the most fiercely sought after gold. Racers wanted to win the gold so badly they made modifications to their aircraft that stretched the rules as far as possible in hopes of making their plane faster than any of the others.

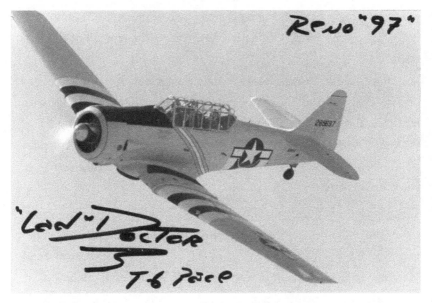

Reno '97.
Compliments of Laird Doctor

"Eddie Van Fossen modified an airplane that was just the fastest damn T-6," remembered Lad. "He was a crop duster and knew about round edges, sharp turns and flying low. He ran a very professional program and smartly made one modification to his airplane at a time. Van Fossen flew to five Gold Cup Championships at the Reno Air Races and set several speed records.

"Others wanted the gold so badly they would make ten or more changes at a time to the aircraft, which made it very difficult to know which modification helped and which one hurt the program. The Reno race was an expensive hobby and not for the faint of heart because it is a financially losing thing for everybody."

The desire to win felt by Indy car drivers was the same adrenalin rush felt by T-6 pilots. They wanted nothing less than to win!

"At one point, taping was a big deal," remembered Lad. "It changed the drag and made the aircraft slicker. We taped the canopy closed from the inside with clear packing tape. Of course, if you need to jump out, it was going to be a bitch. Oh, let me start tearing the tape off of this damn thing."

The crowd couldn't see the entire race, so they relied on the announcers to be their eyes. The unlimited race course was about eight miles long, with laps around huge pylons. Judges stood below the markers and looked up through the pylons. If they could see any part of the airplane as the pilot cut the corner, he was penalized. A judge waved a large checkered flag when a plane crossed the finish line.

The pylons were 50 feet tall, and a pilot's head could not drop below the top of the pylon without being penalized. The Unlimited races consisted mainly of modified WWII fighters—P-51 Mustangs, F-8F Bearcats, and Hawker Sea Furys, and could reach speeds of 500 miles per hour.

"The T-6 races had an extra flair of excitement with an emphasis on flying in very close proximity to other aircraft and pilot skill rather than raw horsepower," explained Lad. "The T-6 averages about 220-230 miles per hour on the five mile course at Reno."

Each Condor flew his personal T-6 to Reno, raced it and returned home in it. This turned into "let's have a race team and what are the rules?" That turned into "let's see if we can get around the rules. What engine or mechanical modifications can be made? What if we polish the aircraft?" This turned it into serious racing instead of a weekend of fun.

Each racer had a specific place in line behind the pace plane. The airplanes were lined up side-by-side like a horse race. When the green flag dropped, they were off to the races. Their place in line had been determined by their time from the qualifying race held at the beginning of the week. Everyone wanted the shortest distance, so when the race began, pilots rushed for the inside lane, creating a level of danger.

Lad offered to polish Charlie Beck's airplane in exchange for the opportunity to be a part of his team. If Charlie was double-booked, Lad raced the T-6 while Charlie raced Howard Keefe's P-51D.

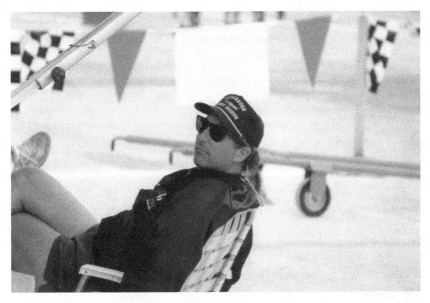

At Reno wearing a Cavanaugh Museum cap.
Compliments of Laird Doctor

Charlie Beck, a decorated World War II pilot, received many awards during his service, including the Distinguished Flying Cross, Air Medal (seven times), Unit Citation, and numerous other distinguished recognitions. He and Bill Statler, a retired engineer from the Lockheed Skunk Works program, built a racing plane that could break numerous records. The Super 6 was built from scratch and totally unique. Per their agreement, Bill Statler designed the plane and Charlie fronted most of the cost, if not all of it. Charlie was extremely wealthy. He lived in Laurel Canyon with his wife, Pat, whose father was Harry Miller, a man who designed and built engines that won the Indianapolis 500 nine times. Other cars using his engines won three more times.

Lad entered a "lean to" building, a very narrow shed located inside a large hanger at Van Nuys Airport.

"Here it is!" Charlie announced.

"The airplane was in the development stage," said Lad. "It was a tight fit. It would be like working in a one-car garage with a car in there."

Charlie studied Lad as he inspected the plane. "Would you consider being my backup pilot at the Reno Air Races in this plane?" he asked.

"Hell yeah," Lad said.

"What do you think about the airplane so far?"

Lad turned to the plane.

"I would like your input. If you find anything wrong with Statler's design, please let me know. I have a lot of money riding on this plane."

Lad looked inside. "Charlie, for crying out loud," he said. "This is supposed to be a race plane. You have too many bells and whistles in this damn airplane. Simple is better and certainly lighter. Less weight more thrust. There are gauges everywhere."

They had started with an AT-6 Airframe, a Pratt and Whitney R2800 engine with a homemade prototype monocoque tail with added tubing for strength.

"No jigs?" Lad asked. Jigs are needed to hold and align a structure during construction for a high degree of accuracy. Lad then looked at the wings. "Damn, these things aren't right," he told Charlie.

"In airplanes there are some things you do to counteract other forces that the airplane does by itself," Lad explained. "They weren't doing it that way. They were just eyeballing it and building this thing."

"Charlie, they need to fix this," he told Beck. "The aerodynamics are going to be weird."

"There is an old saying in aviation," said Lad. "If it looks good, it'll fly good. This airplane looked terrible. It was ugly."

"Charlie, I don't know about this," Lad told him. "The leading edge of one wing looks significantly different than the other. And I don't mean design twists. Just different."

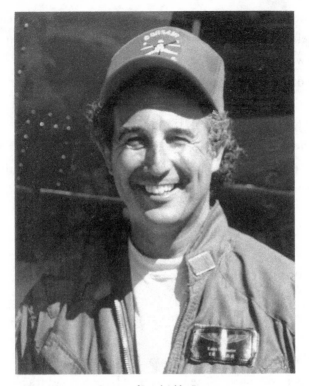

Courtesy of Laird Ashley Doctor.

Lad walked over to Bill Statler and said, "Gee, the engineering is so fascinating. I wish I had been more interested when I was in school. It's amazing that this little piece of steel is going to hold this entire airplane."

"Oh, that's a very special type of steel," Bill replied.

"It's just amazing. It has that huge engine up there that weighs a thousand pounds, the fuel tank and all the other weight on that little piece of steel … simply amazing," replied Lad.

When Lad turned to Bill, bangs and pings suddenly echoed through the building. The entire airplane fell to the ground.

"Fortunately, the landing gear went down and the plane fell on it," said Lad.

"So much for engineering," Lad said under his breath.

111

Charlie had asked for Lad's feedback and he gave him plenty. Many times, their corrective action plan seemed just as scary. Some of Lad's concerns were ignored.

"We don't have time to worry about this or that," Bill would say.

"Sometime later, the airplane was moved to Mojave," said Lad. "And with a 50 foot wing span, it wasn't an easy task."

Charlie and Lad had a lot of experience moving airplanes and knew the tail wheel would be heavy. Their plan was for both to lift the tail as a third person shoved a dolly underneath.

They got under the tail.

"Charlie, you ready?" asked Lad.

"Ready," replied Charlie.

"One, two, three, lift."

"Holy moly I thought the whole airplane was going to flip over," remembered Lad. "There was no weight in the tail. One person could have easily lifted it."

"Charlie, something is wrong with this airplane," said Lad. "You know it as well as I do. You've picked up your AT-6 a lot and it's a hell of a lot heavier than this damn thing. This is wrong."

Charlie agreed.

Finally, in 1978, several years past the promised delivery date, the plane was scheduled to fly. At the Mojave Airport, Champaign bottles were placed on ice and Bill Statler opened one and began celebrating as soon as the plane took off.

"Statler and crew had decided the *Super 6* was going to fly on its first flight and it was going to be wonderful," Lad said.

Joe Guthrie, the test pilot and a friend of Bill Statler, knew what he was doing. His military accomplishments were numerous and he was highly recognized.

Lad listened as Statler explained to Joe that the tail should lift at about 85 miles per hour and the airplane would leave the ground somewhere around 130 to 140 mph. "It's a prototype, a one-off airplane without computers. But everything should be fine," Bill promised.

"Go for it, test pilot!" thought Lad.

As the airplane started down the runway, Bill and the construction crew were already toasting the first flight. But Lad and Charlie weren't ready to celebrate. They watched as Guthrie took off with a much slower rotation than expected, and the Super 6 pitched up to an extremely nose-high attitude.

"Charlie, he has full right rudder, full right aileron, full forward stick and the airplane is in a very high pitch attitude, making a left turn," Lad said.

"This is not a comfortable scene," he explained. "To anyone who has any knowledge of aerodynamics and airplanes, this looks like if he had an ejection seat, it would have been used."

Lad watched, horrified.

"We heard the power reduce and the power reduce and the power go up and the power reduce and the airplane continues in this attitude, making this left-hand turn. This thing is in a high-alpha, gentle left turn, almost like a helicopter."

The gentle left turn became a 180 degree turn back to the runway. As Joe Guthrie further reduced power, the nose began to pitch down a bit. Guthrie managed to get the Super 6 on the ground. Once stopped, he climbed out of the airplane and said, "I will never set foot in that piece of shit again. Get somebody else."

"There was no question Joe Guthrie had skill," said Lad. "You certainly don't get through something like that without a little bit of luck on your shoulder, too."

"That thing leaped off the ground at 90 miles an hour," stated Guthrie. "It wanted to go straight up and turn left. I put everything in to stop the turn. I had to nurse it around and back to the runway, and before it turned past the runway, because I couldn't stop it from turning."
"He did a hell of a job getting the plane back on the runway without any damage," said Lad. "A miracle. An absolute miracle."

"The first flight of the *Super 6* is great! Hot damn," Lad said, laughing.

"And it's the scariest looking picture. As you watch all of the input, he is maybe 50 feet off the ground and you see the aileron and rudder, elevator input and attitude. That plane is not going anywhere. Guthrie's knowledge as a test pilot saved his rear end. To say he was angry would be an understatement to the feeling that he got stuffed into that thing. I am out of here. Give me my money.

"Charlie wasn't happy either, and out of a lot of money," Lad said. "Later, after the Super 6 was reconfigured, Bill Statler hired Skip Holm to test it. It is standard practice for a test pilot to confer with the initial pilot before he steps in the cockpit. One could make a pretty safe assumption that, during Joe Guthrie's conversation with Skip Holm, he was told, 'Don't fly that plane!! You're crazy if you do!' Within seconds, Holm destroyed the plane by sending it over on its nose, and sadly it appeared calculated and deliberate."

§

Sometime later, Lad found himself in a bit of a bind. He needed a new transmission for his car, but could not afford it. He knew that Don's father owned a transmission shop, but needed the telephone number. As a boy, Lad's cousin, Larry, lived within walking distance so Lad knew many of Larry's friends, Don included.

While at the shop, his cousin asked, "So what do you do at the bank?"

"Large commercial loans, mostly," Lad replied.

"Well, I am a large borrower," Larry said.

"Oh yeah, which bank?"

"Independence Bank."

"We're a little bit larger than Independence Bank," said Lad.

Larry discussed a development project that his company, Woodland Construction, wanted to pursue, but needed a large loan to move forward. Lad saw value in the project, but as he worked on a loan package for his cousin, he said, "You need someone in this deal that has some horsepower to improve your financial statement."

"I have a guy," replied Larry. "But he is going to want a big chunk of my project."

"Well 50% of 50 million, over several years, is a lot better than zero of 50 million," advised Lad.

Later, Larry called and said that Frank Arciero had agreed to co-sign. Due to the size of the loan, Lad discussed the situation with higher-ups in the bank.

"A man by the name of Frank Arciero has agreed to back the loan," Lad said.

"Frank Arciero! Give him anything he wants," replied the bank executive. "But know that Arciero is a very busy man."

At the loan closing, Lad had meticulously placed all the needed paperwork around the conference room table so all involved could easily walk around the table, sign the papers and go about their business. After gathering up the paperwork, Lad noticed that Frank Arciero had accidently missed signing the actual note.

"Let's meet at my office and I'll sign it," replied Arciero after Lad discovered the missed signature.

"Wow! Arciero's office was breathtaking!" remembered Lad. It was huge. An Italian village was painted along one wall and Lad's childhood memories flashed before his eyes when they stepped inside an adjacent building filled with race cars.

Larry later convinced Lad to work for him by promising him that he would make a sizeable return on investments as the Assistant Foreman of residential, office space and shopping center projects, as well as other projects Larry and Arciero had partnered in. However, Larry did not stand by his word.

"What am I going to do now that I left the bank?" Lad asked. With a family to take care of, his cousin had left him worse off than if he had stuck with the bank.

Larry replied with an offer of a salaried position, which was a far cry from the return on the other investments he had promised, but Lad felt stuck and accepted the job. Before long, Lad was doing the foreman's work too. So Larry fired the foreman and gave the job to Lad. But without the equivalent salary.

"I was pissed off," said Lad.

§

Cars whipped by in both directions. Between the passing cars, Lad peddled up the hill with unheard-of speed. He had traveled over 12 of the 35 miles it would take before he would reach Simi Valley to the Valley of Los Angeles where he was the scheduled speaker. He was strong and the heat never broke his rhythm. Wearing a T-shirt and bicycle shorts, Lad raised himself off the seat of his ten-speed, forging on to the Saturday meeting.

In sync with every turn of the pedals, Lad repeated over and over, "God … you … can't … make … it … tough … enough. I can take it! You … can't … make … it … tough … enough. You … can't … make … it … tough … enough." 35 miles of anger.

"I was pissed off at the world in general," Lad remembered.

Chapter 13

The Godfather

"Sir, this is Laird Doctor. I don't know if you remember me?"

On the other end of the call was Frank Arciero.

"I do," he replied.

"Would you help me obtain a bank interview?" Lad asked.

"Everything Arciero touched turned to gold," Lad remembered. "And bank presidents loved him."

"Come work for me," said Arciero. "But don't leave your cousin's business just yet. I need your assistance with a couple of issues involving some dealings with Larry's company. Would you be willing to help me?"

Lad agreed.

"I was told that Frank Arciero thought that I was a very loyal person," Lad said.

Arciero immediately put Lad in charge of a large project in California City and entrusted him with the responsibility of reporting the financial honesty of various partners.

At this time, Lad was active in both politics and community service. He assisted Frank Visco, chairman of the California Republican Party for "Bush 41" and Governor Pete Wilson. Visco placed Lad on several committees, and because Lad had to travel to Sacramento every other week, Admiral Hacker, Chairman of the Veterans Affairs, offered to escort Lad, which brought him even closer to war veterans and heroes.

"I nearly tripped on my beard when I met Bob Cardenas," Lad marveled. "You're that guy." Robert Cardenas piloted the B-29 that launched the X-1, an experimental jet designed to shatter the sound barrier.

Lad enjoyed working alongside Charles Kaman, creator of the K-225 Mixmaster, a helicopter with intermeshing rotor blades, like a mixer.

"Charles was a very nice guy to work with politically," said Lad.

§

"You're kidding me," said Terry Otis. "Just like that? All those houses?" Lad had a reputation for hiring the best contractors and never cutting any corners.

"We hit it off immediately and became serious friends," said Terry.

Lad had just given Terry a huge contract for a development project in California. Later, as Terry welded inside a wall, the black tarpaper caught fire. "I had not worked for Lad long and barely knew him when he walked around the corner and called me, Terry the Torch. And the name has stuck for 35 years."

"Terry reciprocated and began calling me, Laddie," said Lad. "Never knowing that it had once been my childhood moniker."

§

"I had a really good deal," said Lad. "The Baron, one of Arciero's airplanes, stayed with me in Paso Robles, California." As Arciero, Lad and another company pilot walked from the plane, Frank stopped, turned around and asked, "What are you two talking about?

"Airplanes," Lad answered.

"What do you do for a living?" Arciero asked.

"I build houses," Lad replied

"Yes! That is how you make your living," said Frank. "So you talk about lumber. You talk about plumbing. You talk about that kind of stuff. You don't talk about airplanes."

§

"Would you like to fly down to Orange County with me to pick up Frank?" Lad asked.

"Heck yeah!" Terry replied.

"It was a spectacular flight," remembered Terry. "The skies were crystal clear and we listened to radio communications as we flew out of LAX."

"Wait until you meet Frank," said Lad. "He sounds like the Godfather."

"Holy Criminy!" exclaims Terry. "He sounded exactly like him!"

"On the return trip, there was a six-foot ceiling in Paso Robles," remembered Terry. "I could not believe it. Lad made such a perfect touchdown. It was unreal."

It was as if he had been groomed his whole life for this job. A contractor gig with the perks of flying and frequenting the Indy races.

§

Katie walked with her father down the side of the Indy race track amongst the cars and the racers. And, most importantly to a teenager, in front of half a million people who probably wished they were in her shoes. "Profiling was what the teenagers called it," said Lad. "When they had an opportunity to stand in front of a crowd and look important. At this moment, Katie was enjoying supreme profiling."

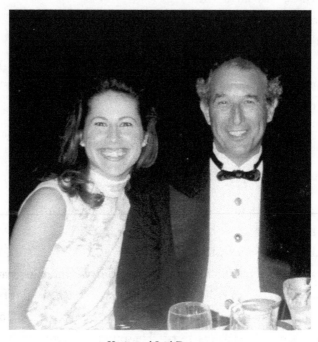

Katie and Lad Doctor.
Compliments of Laird Doctor

Lad's family had been in the race car business since he was a small boy, so it was a way of life for him.

"As Katie and I waited in Frank's office, Mario Andretti walked in with his son," remembered Lad. Katie was getting a taste of what her father's childhood had been like.

"Frank Arciero Jr., 'Butch,' and I had attended a few races together," said Lad. "Butch restored and raced many of his father's cars."

§

"It is in my brain," said Lad.

In addition to heating and air conditioning, Lad's friend, Terry Otis, was a licensed boxing promoter for the state of California. And though he had witnessed many fights, it would be this fight that impressed both Terry and Lad above all others. On November 22, 1986, at the Las Vegas Hilton in Paradise, Nevada, Lad and Terry attended the WBC Heavyweight Championship between Trevor Berbick and Mike Tyson, billed as Judgment Day.

"This was the most unbelievable experience I had ever experienced in my life," said Terry. "Mike Tyson is roughly 20 years old and is fighting for the heavyweight championship of the world and we are there! I am in the aisle seat and Mike Tyson is coming down our aisle! It sends chills down my back just thinking about it. He is right there! Wow! That was the aura of that guy."

"I remember clear as day," said Lad. "I don't think he was robed, and there was a mob of people around him."

"We were in total awe," said Terry.

"And he had a look in his eye," said Lad. "I thought holy moly, this fight is over with. Oooh man." Tyson ended the fight in the second round, hitting Berbick with a right to the body, then a left hook to the head. Berbick attempted to get up twice, but the referee called the fight on a technical knockout. Tyson won, becoming the undisputed heavyweight champion.

"He knocked Trevor out," said Terry. "It was the most unbelievable thing I had ever seen." Being in the business, he had seen a lot of boxing matches in his profession, but this one was the one he could never forget.

"Don King did not take care of Mike Tyson like Cus D'Amato did," said Terry. "When Cus D'Amato died, Tyson's whole life changed."

§

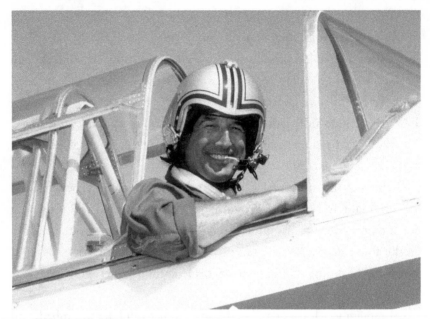

November 22, 1986 at Reno. "The plane I used as a pace plane.
This airplane belonged to Jimmy Good from Casper, Wyoming."
Compliments of Laird Doctor

"It was a big 'ol gaggle," said Lad. He led a procession of about 50 AT-6's in a long caravan across the sky for the 50th anniversary of the AT-6. It started on the west coast with additional AT-6's joining the caravan as they flew across the country. "The FAA stayed in constant correspondence since the corridor up the Hudson was so thin."

Lad flew in many memorial celebrations around the world.

§

July 23, 1987, Dorothy and Lad divorced after 17 years of marriage. "Military is pretty hard on families," Lad lamented.

Katie was their priority and they stayed in constant communication for her sake.

Chapter 14

Plant 42

Lad and Colonel Mario Cafiero served on a committee to create community awareness of the significance in keeping Air Force Plant 42 in Palmdale, California viable. Development was squeezing the base out.

"All the major airplane companies in the United States had facilities there," explained Lad.

> *Attraction to the area for the aviation companies was the main runways and ramp/taxi space. The main runway 07/25 is 12,000 in length and is the strongest runway in the world, built to withstand an 8.3 Earthquake. (Plant 42 is near the San Andreas Fault). It also has some of the best firefighting equipment in the United States and the fire crews are some of the best trained in the country.[21]*

Cafiero would later say, "Commanding Plant 42 was my favorite assignment."

Col. Mario Cafiero was one of Air Force Plant 42's most visible commanders. As Plant 42 commander from June 22, 1988 to July 27, 1990, Cafiero sparred with city officials and developers to ward off development under flight paths and convinced the Air Force to rescind a decision to sell off the installation

"Aside from the location and outstanding community support, being the commander of the Air Force Production Flight Test Installation during such an exciting time in its history made that assignment stand out among so many wonderful Air Force opportunities," said Cafiero.

"Palmdale is the birthplace of so many initial production aircraft, and I was fortunate enough to experience that firsthand, particularly with the B-2, the space shuttle orbiter, and a range of exciting modification and test programs." [22]

In the effort to educate the community about the importance of Air Force Plant 42, Lad volunteered to give local high school students the opportunity of a lifetime: a ride in an AT-6. This began an annual career event called "Salute to Youth." The students were brought in through a back gate to distance them from the classified areas.

"If the children had realized the history they were looking at . . . ." said Lad. "We had the SR-71, the experimental X29, the F117, and more." The use of these Air Force assets came about through a request by Cafiero. Dave Bruce, the owner of the AT-6 used for the career event, asked Lad if it would be possible to get all three planes in a picture. Lad passed the request onto Cafiero, and the next day tractors moved the F-117 Nighthawk and the SR-71 Blackbird with the AT-6 Texan and Dave Bruce got his picture.

Lad received the 1990 Developer of the Year award for structuring an agreement between local school districts and developers while bringing awareness of the importance of Plant 42.

§

While living in Palmdale, Lad became involved in politics. William J. "Pete" Knight, a decorated pilot in the Vietnam War, was the first Mayor for the City of Palmdale to be popularly elected. Colonel Knight, Lad, numerous test pilots, military veterans, and others, attended a fund raiser in downtown Los Angeles for Mayor Knight's aspirations of becoming a state senator representing California's 17th Senate District.

As a California state Senator, William Knight will always be remembered for authoring Proposition 22, the Knight Initiative, which defined marriage as a union only between a man and a woman.

Lad participated in many political fundraisers, but this one was special. William J. Knight was a friend, hero, smart business man, and possessed high moral convictions that no social pressure could burst. The public must have felt the same because the William J. (Pete) Knight High School, home of the Knight Hawks, would open its doors to freshmen in Palmdale, California, in August 2003.

Pete Knight's speed record in an X-15 hypersonic rocket-powered fixed wing aircraft—4,520 miles per hour—has never been broken. Two spacecraft were named in his honor as an astronaut, White Knight One and White Knight Two. He was one of only five pilots to earn their Astronaut Wings by flying an aircraft in space. The Pete Knight Veterans Home of California was yet another honor. Years later, Knight was memorialized at The Aerospace Walk of Honor in Lancaster, California.

Lad took Pete Knight for a ride down memory lane in an AT-6.

"I really enjoyed the flight because Pete was most certainly a consummate aviator," said Lad.

§

Lad had now attended the Reno Air Races for 16 years. As he and Ray Shutty, an excellent fixed wing pilot, stood in the FAA check line to prove their biannual flight review was up-to-date, they were not alone. Every pilot who planned to race that year stood in that line for the same purpose.

"Hey Lad," a pilot yelled from the front of the line. "Will you sign off my biannual?"

"Yeah," Lad said with a laugh. "I'll come up there." This would be a recurring theme. "I knew they had completed the needed requirements."

"'Lad!' yelled Ray Shutty, with all his mega flying hours. The FAA officers are laughing and look up, 'Lad, you're biannual is out of date.'"

"Somebody stop Ray!" yelled Lad. "Ray! Get back in here and sign my biannual."

"These guys are out of their minds," said the FAA officers.

§

While at the Annual International Council of Air Shows (ICAS) in Las Vegas, Charles Hutchins walked over to the AT-6 Racing Association table and informed Lad that a friend was looking for someone to run his new Aircraft Museum and fly his warbirds in air shows.

Lad was intrigued. Charlie gave Jim Cavanaugh Lad's contact information and an interview took place over the phone. Since Katie was preoccupied with college, Lad took the job. He left an extraordinary life behind in California and moved to Addison, Texas, to run the Cavanaugh Flight Museum. Lad continued to be a very valuable person at Reno and he tried to get Jim Cavanaugh interested in the Reno Races, but Cavanaugh never found any interest.

"To be honest," said Lad. "I really didn't want to leave Frank Arciero."

How could any profession even come close to the excitement he had while working for Frank? However, Lad would be more than pleasantly surprised. In fact, Jim and Arlene Cavanaugh asked him, "What is it going to take to get you out of here? Stick dynamite in your office chair or something?"

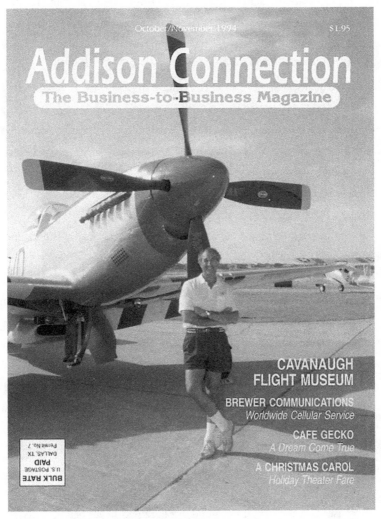

1993, Lad at home as the director and chief pilot of the Cavanaugh Flight Museum, located at Addison Airport, in Dallas, Texas.

Compliments of Laird Doctor

"Well if I had a weekend off," replied Lad. "I would probably search for interesting airplanes. You have the best collection around, right here. And that is how I felt. To me, the museum was a labor of love. I enjoyed being there. I had the same emotional feelings as Jim had for reasons of having the museum. And I truly developed an emotional feeling for the museum and the aircraft there. That was my life."

Established in 1993, the Cavanaugh Flight Museum promotes aviation education, research and American aviation heritage. It also provides aircraft restoration, operates and maintains flying aircraft, and maintains and displays historically-significant vintage aircraft. And standing next to one of Cavanaugh's planes was a wax dummy dressed in Lad's original flight suit.

Lad worked seven days a week, almost 24 hours a day.

"Take a vacation," Cavanaugh ordered.

"I was never going to get rich working there," said Lad. "But the perks! Those made it worth it."

Lad's family and friends were in California, but he remembered one individual from the Reno Races who lived in the Dallas area named Linda Finch. He gave her a call, and after a two-year friendship, they began dating. In 1995, shortly after graduating from college, Katie moved to Dallas and in with her father.

During this time Linda Finch was restoring a Lockheed Model 10E Electra, the 15th of only 149 Model 10's that Lockheed had built, and only one of two still in existence. Her aspiration was to restore the Electra to exactly mirror Amelia Earhart's plane, and fly the same flight path around the world on the 60th anniversary of Earhart's infamous flight. However, politics would get involved.

"Because Amelia Earhart's original airplane had never been located," said Lad, "Pratt & Whitney resolved with the FAA that the engines were destroyed, allowing Linda to reissue Earhart's data plates on her newly-built engines."

After numerous discussions with the FAA, they finally capitulated to Lad's reasoning and allowed Linda to paint Amelia Earhart's tail number, N16020, on her plane as long as Linda's registration number was painted under the tail. That way, if Amelia's plane ever surfaced, there would not be two aircraft with the same tail number. During Amelia Earhart's time, the N was the beginning of a five-digit registration number. Today, people can personalize their registration number. Instead of the letter N, Lad's friend Clay Lacy used his initials, CL, as part of his number.

Linda asked Lad to fly around the world with her, but he refused. "I'm not qualified," he told her.

Because of the significance of the flight, the news media blanketed the skies with helicopters and private planes, hoping to see her fly off.

"Every news agency around the world was in the sky," said Lad, and because of this, he agreed to fly the first leg for her, but no one knew that Lad was in the cockpit, too. But it would be the only leg he flew. The rest was history: starting on March 17, 1997, Finch successfully flew around the world following Amelia Earhart's planned route as closely as possible, flying 26,000 miles in 73 days.

"I wasn't supposed to get any publicity, so I was already slouched down in the co-pilot seat when the public watched Linda climb into the plane wearing a tailor-made flight suit to match Amelia Earhart's attire worn that day 60 years ago. After that leg, she was on her own. Linda's trip was quite an accomplishment."

§

Cavanaugh Flight Museum was the catalyst that brought Lad together with the many war heroes he idolized. "Wow what a phenomenal experience," said Lad. "To meet all those guys and girls."

He walked in the door dressed in his full regalia—a retired Russian General and MIG-15 test pilot, complete with a translator. The General did not come to America to see war planes. This Russian was a Christian and was a special guest speaker at an area church. Through his translator, he asked Lad if he could return that evening for the Christmas Carols and party.

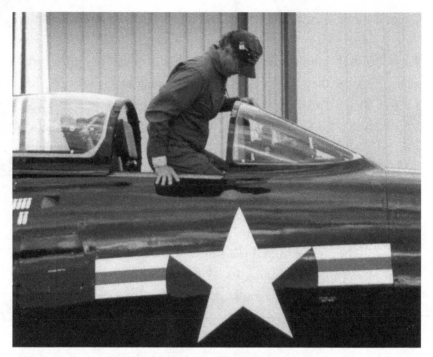

Grumman F9F Panther.
Compliments of Laird Doctor

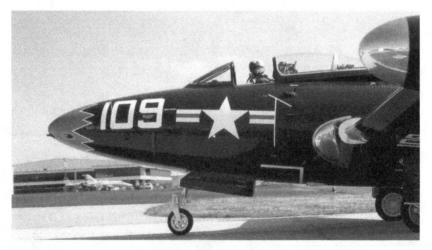

Grumman F9F Panther.
Compliments of Laird Doctor

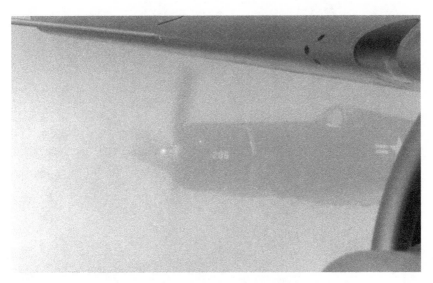

Flying his favorite plane, the Vought F4U Corsair.
Compliments of Laird Doctor

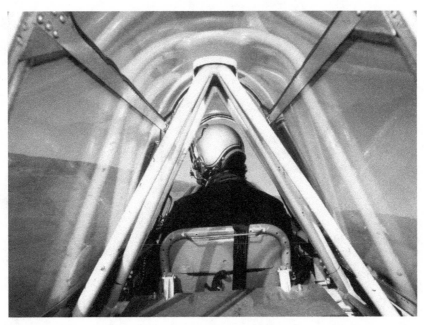

Lad at the helm of an AT-6 Texan.
Compliments of Laird Doctor

ADOLF GALLAND
GENERALLEUTNANT A.D.

EIFELWEG 26
53424 REMAGEN
TEL. (02228) 7171

1. Februar 1995

Cavanaugh Flight Museum;Inc
4572 Claire Chennault
Dallas, Texas 75248
U.S.A.

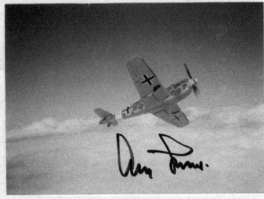

Dear Mr. Laird,

Thank you for your letter and invitaion, dated 22nd of December 94.

I am sorry to say, not beeing able to be your guest at the 50th
Anniversary of V.E.Day. My reduced health condition doesn't allow me
to make long travels.

I wish you a very pleasant and special event in May.

Best regards
Sincerely

Adolf Galland

It hate
I have flown the Me 109 with Rolls.
Royce engine 1980 in Spain. The
restricted visenbility is lousy.
A. P.

RECEIVED
FEB 10 1995

Adolf Galland, WWII German Luftwaffe General and Flying Ace.
He died one year after writing this letter to Lad.
Compliments of Laird Doctor

One after another they came. Throughout the years, Lad would have the opportunity to come face to face with those he held with high regard. One of these was Keith Ferris, a valued artist whose work adorns the halls of the Pentagon and the National Air and Space Museum. He gave Lad a portrait of a C-17 Globemaster III cargo aircraft. Keith was a 50-year veteran of the Air Force, whose primary job was recreating aircraft while in the testing phase.

On May 5, 1995, Lad was mingling with the military's finest at Cavanaugh's. It wasn't just another date on the calendar to them, though. It was the 50th Anniversary of V.E. Day or Victory in Europe Day. They had fought in World War II and had smelled death at their door. To America's heroes, it marked the formal Allied acceptance of Nazi Germany's unconditional surrender of its armed forces, ending World War II in Europe.

Working at the Cavanaugh Flight Museum was the perfect job. Lad appreciated the people and the planes that stood for freedom. One day his phone started to ring.

"Will you fly my plane?" the voice asked.

Lad not only had the opportunity to fly Cavanaugh's historic aircraft, but also those from other museums as well. He began receiving numerous requests from owners across the country to fly all kinds of planes and report issues found. He was participating in 20 to 24 airshows a year. He flew so often that the FAA sliced out the "waiting game" if he needed anything.

"Every weekend I was someplace flying and meeting pilots, which led to more and more flying and more and more opportunities to fly. It truly was, for me, a wonderful job. I know at the end of the first year, when the anniversary came around, I had worked, without noticing it, seven days a week.

§

"As Connie Edwards, who had one of the world's finest collections of WWII-era warplanes, taxied his Catalina at Oshkosh, he yells out the window, 'Hey, Lad! Want a beer?' He drops a beer from the cockpit, which is pretty high off the ground," remembered Lad.

"I'm parking. Come aboard," he yelled.

"That thing was littered with cans," remembered Lad.

Chapter 15

Lad Doctor, Stunt Pilot, Me 109

Add stunt pilot to Lad's list of accomplishments. Tuskegee Airmen, the 1995 movie starring Laurence Fishburne, Cuba Gooding Jr., John Lithgow, and Malcolm-Jamal Warner also starred Lad Doctor and Cavanaugh's own Messerschmitt Me 109.

To simulate shooting down a P-51 Mustang, Lad was instructed to follow closely on its tail.

"Lower! No, LOWER!" barked the movie's director.

"The directors of the Tuskegee Airmen wanted a shot of the 109 coming straight at the camera," said Lad. "Fly lower!" they insisted.

Lad discussed the situation with the P-51 pilot. Lad was at the disadvantage because he was instructed to fly below the P-51.

"Let's try this out before they shoot the scene," Lad said. "I will fly under and behind you. When I say, 'no lower,' note the altitude because that will be your altitude during the shoot. I will jerk around to give the chase-and-shoot effect."

Lad came down low, just like he was instructed, and when he did the cameraman fell off the ladder.

"We were going to hit the damn ladder. They wanted a head shot of this P-51 with me close behind and lower. He got his shot. Nothing but propeller. The gun shots fired from the Messerschmitt were created with graphics and small, blinking lights. A costume? What do I need a costume for? 'Well, because you are flying a P-51 or a 109,' they said. But all you will see is my head. What do you care what clothes I have on?" Lad replied.

The pilots would not be in the movie. The actors sat in parked planes, twisting and turning to appear as the real deal. Lad showed the crew a pair of goggles and a jacket he had that resembled the period. They liked it and that is what he wore. But the P-51 pilots were in full makeup.

"Makeup!" yelled the director. "Fix their makeup!"

"We were there three or four days," said Lad. He was impressed with the pilots and knew most of them. The studio paid $3,500 a day for the plane. "The weather in Muskogee, Oklahoma, was really crappy," said Lad.

"Lad, Can you fly today?" they asked.

"Nope. Not in this wind," Lad replied. "It was blowing!"

When the rain finally stopped, Lad figured he could work around the puffy clouds.

"Cut!" the director yelled. "You're flying too fast."

This time, they wanted Lad to dive toward the cameraman, but at an angle. That was close to impossible because behind and to the left of the camera man was a hanger. As Lad flew over the camera man, the hanger to his left would be hard to miss. Lad took off, pulled up and put the power on, rolled in and started downhill.

"Cut!" they yelled. "You're flying too fast."

"Slower meant less throttle," said Lad. "A Merlin engine is what this 109 had. If you idle any airplane engine, every few minutes you need to boost the engine to clear out any carbon buildup. It may cough, sputter and backfire, but after you blow out some of the garbage, it will run smoothly. They wanted me to come down so slowly that I was close to idling. The minute I cleared the picture, I flew over the cameraman and just pulled up and put the power on, and when I did the plane coughed. It did not want any power and continued to cough as I was pulling out."

The film crew attempted to contact Lad over the radio.

"Wait a minute," replied Lad. "I have a rough runner and I'm trying to sort out the problem."

"The airport is yours and aid is coming," they replied. "Do you need anything? How is the engine running? What seems to be the problem? Which runway do you want to use?"

"Wait a minute, wait a minute," said Lad. "I have to figure this out first."

The 109 was still banging.

"I don't own this airplane," said Lad. "But I pretty much know what it is. I just need some high power on this engine for a little while."

Lad chose the runway that would offer the most wind to fly into. However, it was the shortest runway too.

"At that point in my learning curve," explained Lad. "I did not know a whole lot about the 109. So landing was an interesting affair."

After he landed, his fellow pilots were extremely impressed. Over the radio he heard, "Nice landing!"

"Wait a minute!" Lad said. "I'm going to open my eyes and take a look."

Out of all the hard work, there was only one little sequence used in the movie. It was that last shot. The one that almost killed Lad and the airplane before it was all over.

§

Sometime later, while Lad was working to get the museum ready for a special event one day, Lad turned to see a gentleman walking towards him. "He wasn't invited, he just happened to walk into Cavanaugh's one day. W-O-W! WOW! This is something!" Lad said as he shook the man's hand.

He wasn't just a Navy Frogman. He was the first allied military soldier at Normandy beach. His job was to locate and defuse underwater mines, fences and traps, clearing the way for the historic invasion.

§

Charlie Bond, the Flying Tiger who had discussed painting the open mouth of a snarling tiger shark on the American Volunteer Group's P-40s with his squadron mates and with Claire Chennault, and whose story of triumph blasted from the radio in the corner when Lad was a baby, was now Lad's esteemed friend.

"Over the years, many have utilized the name *Flying Tigers*," said Lad.

The original Flying Tigers were also known as the AVG, American Volunteer Group. A small group of heroes who, under the command of General Claire Lee Chennault, became members of the Chinese Air Force (not the U.S. Army Air Corps) and heroically fought off the Japanese as they attempted to take over China. After they disbanded, the AVG was gobbled up by the 14th Air Force.

Everyone who served in the 14th Air Force began calling themselves Flying Tigers, and in some ways that diminished the original name. The only Air Force unit that was in fact granted the use of the name *Flying Tigers* by the original AVG was a helicopter unit.

Charlie Bond hosted a Flying Tigers reunion in Dallas in 1996. Every table was adorned with a small flying tiger statue with the signatures of the *Flying Tigers* who had spent the afternoon signing them until their hands gave out. Close to 1,000 appreciative patrons attended, and Charlie and Lad saw to it that at least one Flying Tiger and their spouse was seated at each table. The autographed statues were intended for the Flying Tiger at that table. But someone forgot to tell that to the Flying Tigers. So instead of the Tigers having a keepsake with their comrade's signatures to pass down to their children, they would be taken home by random attendees.

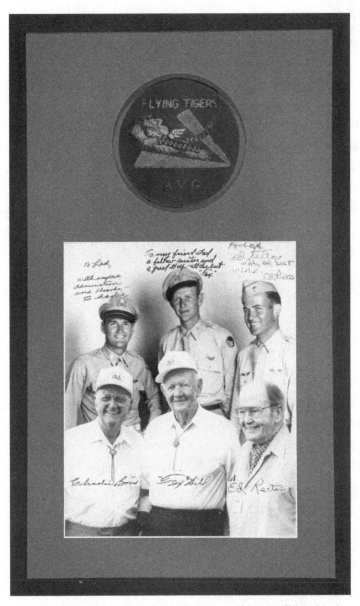

"I was a really close with both Charlie Bond and 'Tex' Hill," said Lad. Charlie had two pictures. The original in their uniforms, and the other was an effort to recreate the original. Lad asked if he could superimpose the two pictures. Charlie said, "No I'll take care of it." "Charlie made four autographed copies. One for each of them and one for me," said Lad.

Compliments of Laird Doctor

"The 1942 Flying Tigers movie starring John Wayne was loosely depictive of reality," said Lad.

Lad took his grandchildren to meet Major General Charlie Bond, United States Air Force, just so they could have a picture with a man who will go down in history as a true hero.

The Flying Tigers, The Condor Club and the Quiet Birdmen were efforts by those who understood, for those who understood, and to educate those who didn't. Lad understood their sacrifices firsthand, appreciated them and was honored to say he was a friend.

And because of all the heroes such as Bond, Lad's commitment to maintaining and educating all of America with the historic aircraft had a special place in his heart few could understand. He maintained the aircraft like no other.

§

Planning was underway for The Blue Angels' 50th anniversary, celebrating the second oldest formal flying aerobatic team in the world, formed on April 24, 1946.

Lad called the Ops office and informed them that Cavanaugh had the only Panther in the world. "If you want me to fly the Panther at the Blue Angels' 50th anniversary," said Lad. "All I would need in return would be a full tank of gas to return home. I would love to be there. I'd cut my arm off to be there."

"Nope," Replied the Ops office. "We can't give you the fuel."

"I don't understand," replied Lad. "You can't give me a bag of gas? It doesn't hold that much."

Sometime later, Lad bumped into a Blue at an airshow.

"You didn't want the F9F Panther at the 50th?" Lad asked.

"I didn't know anything about it," he said.

"Well, I called the base," Lad replied.

"Who did you talk to?" the Blue asked.

"The Ops Officer," said Lad.

"You should have called the Office of the Blue Angels," he said. "It was our show, not the base's. We had to convince them to do the damn show. Fuel! We would have given you fuel and anything else you wanted."

"I called the wrong office," Lad lamented.

But Lad's appreciation for all the men and women who sacrificed for freedom, and his dedication to the maintenance of the aircraft they used, continued to open doors of opportunity to meet heroes that others could only dream of.

§

The pouring rain did not deter 300 enthusiastic customers from packing into a metal hanger at Cavanaugh's for the opportunity to hear and visit with several renowned pilots and dignitaries: Colonel Gabby Gabreski, the highest-scoring ace in WWII; General Frank Blazey; and Florene Miller Watson, among others.

In January, 1943, she became Commanding Officer of the WASP stationed at Love Field, Dallas. In 1944, she served as a test pilot in a highly secretive program to develop radar equipment for planes. By the time the war was over, Florene had flown every type of training, cargo, fighter, and twin and four-engine bomber that the Air Corps used.

"I remember telling myself when I got on the base, well, during the first week, or first few days, with all these men and all the activity that was going on, I told myself, 'You are not going to do or say anything while you're here that you're going to be embarrassed about fifty years from now.' I can go back to all the reunions and everything else, I think, "You don't have anything on me, buddy.... Because I didn't know what the future was going to bring ...."

*"During the years, I have been asked to give many, many WAFS-
WASP WWII presentations ... been inducted into several prestigious
'Hall of Fame' type honors and been featured in newspapers, books
and magazine articles—but the bottom line for me is—What does
my Lord think of me!" said Florene Miller Watson.* [23]

Lad knew firsthand the sacrifices made by these men and women. He
had deep understanding and admiration for them and their planes, and his
appreciation did not go unnoticed—they would give him books, pictures,
letters, cards, and more throughout the years. These aren't museum pieces
bought at an auction, they are historic, personal gifts given to Lad. One
of these is a pin from Chuck Yeager for taking the general's challenge
seriously—Lad had accumulated 2,000 flight hours flying *Young Eagles*.

Another high point in Lad's life: a conversation with Colonel Paul
Warfield Tibbets about Tibbets' historical flight. Colonel Tibbets, the
pilot of all pilots, described his historic trip to deliver the "material," the
first atomic bomb dropped on Japan on August 6, 1945, in the Boeing
B-29 Stratofortress named after Tibbets' mother: *Enola Gay.*

"The B-29 had been stripped of everything," Paul told Lad. "There
wasn't much left in it. I worked closely with the Wright Company making
needed engine modifications. We anticipated a weight issue with that
monstrous bomb in the belly of that B-29, but we were still a little
surprised to find that when we took off, we just hovered a few feet above
the water. I don't think the airplane took off. As we left the Tinian Island
toward Japan, I just raised the wheels out from under."

They skimmed the surface until weight was reduced through the
burning of fuel. Then the weighed-down B-29 holding the weight of
freedom inside its bomb bay floated a little higher, hovered a bit more until
additional fuel burned, then rose to the next level. The stages continued
until they reached 30,000 feet. Taking on less fuel before takeoff was not
an option. Pilot Paul W. Tibbets, Navigator Theodore J. Van Kirk and
Bombardier Thomas W. Ferebee needed to balance the optimum amount
of fuel to maintain speed and make it to Japan and back.

"Since fuel adds weight," said Lad. "Tibbets flew as high as the bomber could go, which wasn't far, then stayed at that altitude until additional fuel was burned, reducing weight and allowing the plane to climb a little bit further. And again, as fuel burned and reduced the weight, they climbed to the next level and this would continue. He had to take one step at a time.

"They had a tremendous amount of information from the extensive tests performed in Alamogordo, New Mexico," said Lad. "But, dropping an 8,818.49-pound atomic bomb from a plane is a little different than dropping it in the desert with props."

"Lad, I have to tell you," Tibbets said, "we had no idea what this thing was going to be like. We did not know how much destruction would be from the bomb."

"I remember Tibbets said their escape plan required a very steep angle of bank, diving and turning," said Lad. "With the enormous weight, they feared the maneuver might tear the wings off of the damn airplane and feared overstressing the B-29 at the crucial time of attempting to escape the blast."

Would the blast affect them? Were they going to be sucked into this? Would they be a part of the explosion? They would have only a certain amount of time to drop it and leave.

"The *Enola Gay* was stressed trying to escape the blast as the cloud rose higher than they were," explained Lad. "They were beating feet to get out of there."

"On August 6, 1943 as the Enola Gay approached the Japanese city of Hiroshima, I fervently hoped for success in the first use of a nuclear type weapon. To me it meant putting an end to the fighting and the consequent loss of lives. In fact, I viewed my mission as one to save lives rather than to take them. The intervening years has brought me many letters and personal contacts with individuals who maintain that they would not be alive today if it had not been for what I did. Likewise, I have been asked in letters and to my face if I was not

conscience-stricken for the loss of life I caused by dropping the first atomic bomb. To those who ask, I quickly reply "NOT IN THE LEAST." Paul W. Tibbets, Brig General USAF, Retired.[24]

"These were childhood names—heroes, legends," said Lad. "That was probably the greatest part of the museum for me: meeting the people."

Chapter 16

The Hero's Return

Paul Tibbets was a special guest for an event held at Cavanaugh Flight Museum. As he signed autographs, his publicist told Lad, "Toward the end of the war, two signatures could get anything they needed from the United States government, President Roosevelt and General Tibbets. If Tibbets wanted something all he had to do was ask and sign his name and somewhere in the United States they would produce it. He was that powerful at one time."

"Oh, and by the way," said the publicist. "Tibbets will be 82 this weekend."

"Oh my gosh!" said Lad. "Paul came down here to sign autographs for a bunch of Texans on his birthday? I can't believe this!"

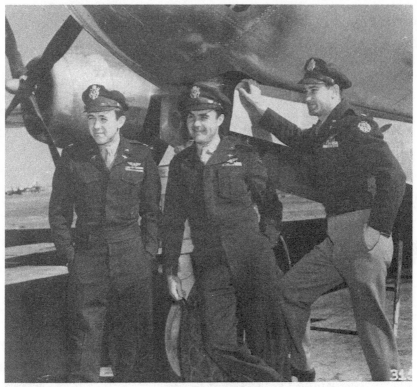

Theodore J. Van Kirk Paul W. Tibbets Thomas W. Ferebee
Navigator Pilot Bombadier

Colonel Paul Warfield Tibbets, the Pilot, Theodore J. Van Kirk,
the Navigator and Thomas W. Ferebee, the Bombardier.
Compliments of Laird Doctor

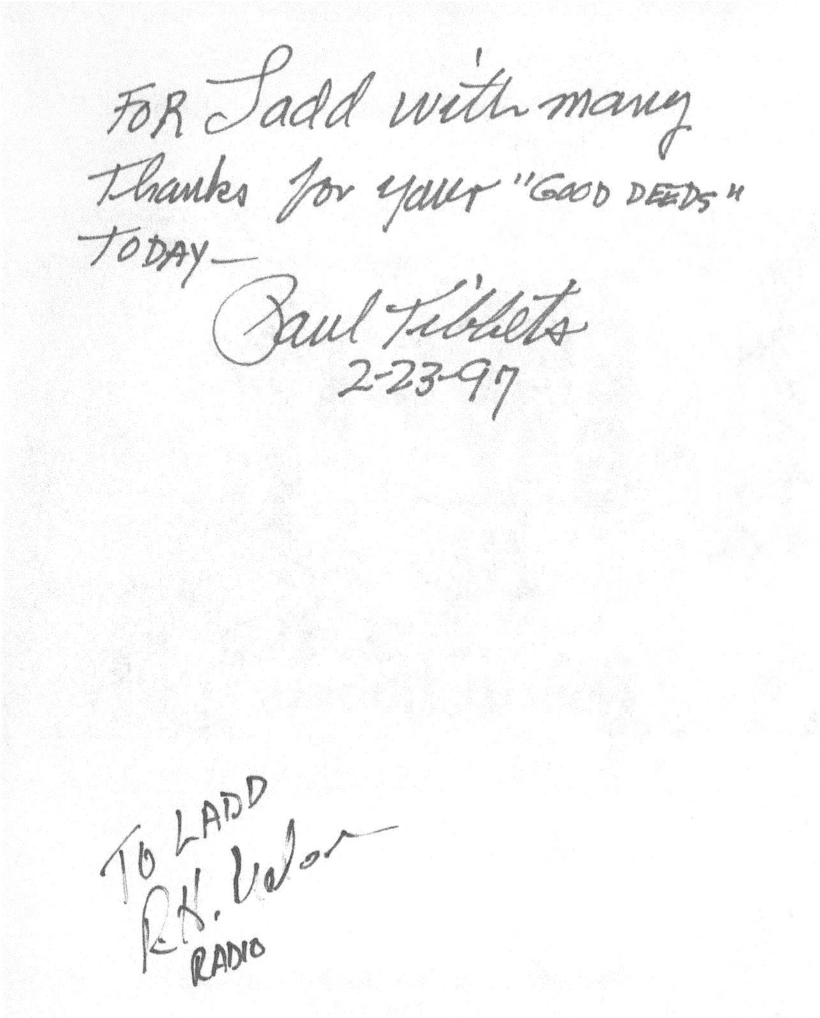

FoR Ladd with many
Thanks for your "GOOD DEEDS"
TODAY—

Paul Tibbets
2-23-97

TO LADD
R.H. Udon
RADIO

Lad immediately put together an impromptu surprise birthday party at a steakhouse on Beltline Road in Addison, Texas. Ray Kenny, a Confederate Air Force board member, ordered and paid for an elaborate birthday cake donning the B-29, complete with propellers and tail number. Major General Charlie Bond, Florene Miller Watson and other famous heroes attended the celebration.

"I can't believe you are down here," Lad told Tibbets. "You've got family and things."

"Paul and I hit it off," remembered Lad. "Like most World War II pilots, he had extreme hearing loss."

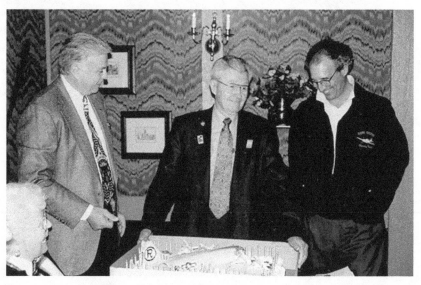

Ray Kenny, Paul Tibbets, Lad and a B-29 birthday cake.
Compliments of Laird Doctor

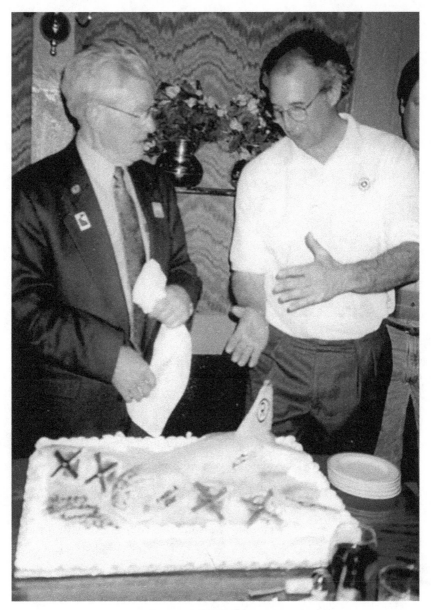

Lad honoring Paul Tibbets with a B-29 birthday cake.
Compliments of Laird Doctor

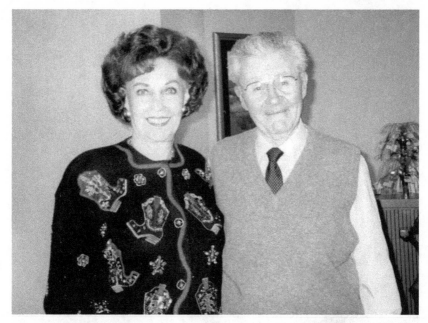

February 23, 1997, two famous World War II heroes: Florene Miller Watson, WASP, flew every kind of aircraft used by the U.S. Army Air Corp., and General Paul Tibbets, pilot of the B-29 *Enola Gay*, which dropped the first atomic bomb on Japan.
Compliments of Laird Doctor

"Sometime later at an event," said Lad, "I remember stepping into the hotel elevator filled with dignitaries and Paul Tibbets: 'Hello General Tibbets.' 'Lad, How the hell are you doing?' replied the General. We chatted until the elevator stopped. The dignitaries in the elevator that day were probably wondering, 'Who is this guy, anyway?'"

And then there was Florene Watson, the young girl with striking beauty who, instead of choosing a "safe" occupation, decided to add value to the war effort with her flying expertise.

Florene Miller Watson

1602 Primrose Lane ◇ Borger, Texas 79007 ◇ (806) 274-3354

March 10, 1997

Dear Lad:

How great it was to see your smiling face again recently. You and your Cavenaugh Museum certainly do have a warm spot in my heart.

Here are a few photos I took of you at the big birthday Tibbets Bash! You look great.

Well here it is the middle of March — the time that you are supposed to fly into the sunset with a compass and see if you can find your way home again. What an undertaking! I hope you find it as rewarding as it should be. Good Luck!

Lad — I want you to know that I certainly do appreciate being included in the Cavenaugh activities and I do thank you for my good dinner and good time at the Tibbets party.

Be careful on your trip. I pray that it will be all you want it to be.

Fondly, Florene

A personal note to Lad from Florene—original
Women's Auxiliary Ferrying Squadron (WAFS).
Compliments of Laird Doctor

"Talk about someone who is tough," said Lad. "While vacuuming, Florene tripped and fell down the stairs, breaking her femur bone. The jagged edges pierced through her skin. When she came to, she began dragging herself toward her office to call 9-1-1. Due to the immense pain, she would sporadically lose consciousness. She wedged herself between the wall and the desk, so that she could pull the phone off of the desk. During the call, she would continue to lose consciousness. When the firefighters and paramedics arrived, she thought, 'Oh great they are here.' But, instead they ran right past her. 'I'm over here,' she yelled."

§

It was February, 17, 1997 at Nellis Air Force Base. "The Chief of Staff of the Air Force and a good friend of mine, General Ronald Fogelman, had the final say as to what would be flown in celebration of the 50th Anniversary of the Air Force," said Lad.

The General told Lad that the Air Force was working with the British to bring their Spitfire to the show. It was his hope to have the Messerschmitt and Spitfire fly together, that is, if he could convince Paul Day, the squadron leader for the British Memorial Flight and Commander of the Tornado 617 Squadron, to bring it from England to Nellis for the celebration. Day agreed.

"The United States Air Force sent a C-5 Cargo Plane to England to transport that very rare and valuable airplane, its crew and spare parts to Nellis Air Force Base," Lad explained. "I flew the Messerschmitt from Addison, Texas, to Nellis at the request of the Air Force Chief of Staff General Ronald Fogelman. The 109 only held 98 gallons of fuel and the engine burns 120 gallons per hour on takeoff. The trip took me five stops over two days," said Lad. "Sitting in the small cockpit of the 109 from Texas to Nellis Air Force Base was painful. The trip was long and uncomfortable and I experienced severe leg cramps. The longest leg of the flight lasted about an hour and a half and my legs were beyond tired. I don't believe I ever flew a leg that long in the 109 again. I was whacked out."

At Nellis, Lad watched the C-5 land with the precious cargo inside. And, he continued to watch as the Spitfire was rolled out the back of it.

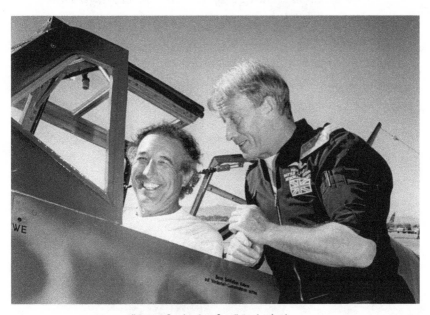

"Can I fly the Spitfire?" Lad asked.
"Nope sorry. But you can sit in it and look around," Paul replied.
Lad Doctor and Commander Paul Day
Compliments of Laird Doctor

"The 109 was parked next to the aircraft Chuck Yeager would fly in the air show because he would be in the flight before us," said Lad. "I had the privilege of meeting General Yeager on several occasions prior to that particular airshow. It was a very prestigious event. The celebration in Las Vegas was not only enjoyable but an immense honor for me to fly in the company of such famous people as Chuck Yeager."

There's no such thing as a natural-born pilot. When I was picked to fly the X-1, it was my duty to fly it, and I did.

October 12, 1944, Lt. Yeager scored five confirmed kills over Bremen, Germany, becoming the first "Ace" in one day.

As group leader, Lt. Yeager was escorting B-24 bombers over Holland when his squadron spotted 22 Bf 109 aircraft. Lt. Yeager spooked one pilot who collided with another, sending both down in flames, continued to shoot down another at 600 yards, then rolled over behind his pursuer to take him out at less than 50 feet. The last pilot went into a steep dive as Lt. Yeager pursued the aircraft, but it could not pull out and barreled into the ground. [25]

In 1947, Yeager became the first pilot confirmed to have exceeded the speed of sound in level flight.

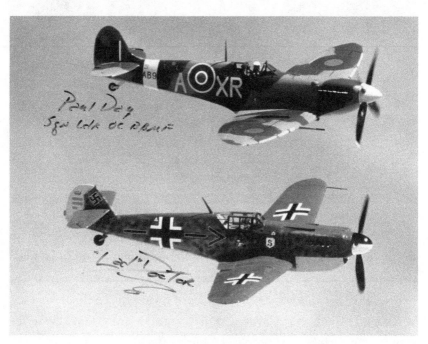

Paul Day, the squadron leader for the British Memorial Flight and Commander of the Tornado 617 Squadron, flying the Spitfire and below Lad flies the Messerschmitt as they make a fly by.
Compliments of Laird Doctor

§

On June 27, 1998, after a somewhat lengthy relationship, and after Lad had an opportunity to first discuss it with his daughter, Katie, Linda Finch and Lad Doctor married.

Chapter 17

Open Heart Surgery

"Lad was a hell of an athlete," said Terry Otis. "He would always kick my butt."

Without Lad realizing it, his father had probably helped develop his athletic ability and the desire to keep moving. Linda and Lad had been married less than a month and everything was going as planned. Lad had spent the weekend representing Cavanaugh's at an event and had looked forward to a relaxing jog to the gym.

"What is that?" thought Lad. The chest pain was so intense, he stopped running. After a few minutes, the pain subsided, and he returned to jogging.

"Wham-o. That hurt!" said Lad. "I walked the rest of the way. After my workout, I walked back to the B.O.Q. However, upon reaching the stairs, I felt fine, so I ran them ten times. I concluded my workout with sit-ups, push-ups and a few other exercises."

Sometime later, he scheduled an appointment with a heart specialist who put him through a battery of tests.

"Walk slowly on the treadmill," the doctor told him. After several minutes he told Lad, "Get off the treadmill and sit down."

"I feel just fine," Lad replied.

"You are going to the hospital and have bypass surgery," was the doctor's response.

On August 2, 1998, the night before his quadruple bypass, as he lay in bed he began to panic.

"Wow, I am having open heart surgery in the morning," he thought. Anxiety took over. "Take me to the hospital," he told Linda. "I need a shot of something to slow me down."

As his anxiety spun out of control, he drove 100 miles per hour to the hospital.

"I'm not supposed to be here for a few hours, but I need something now," he told the nurse at the front desk.

"You're a little anxious are you?" she replied.

"No, I'm a lot anxious," Lad said. "And my body is not going to sustain this much longer."

He was given a room and a shot. The next thing he knew there was a nurse standing beside his bed.

"You need to cough," the nurse told him. "You must cough to rid the build-up in your lungs."

Lad attempted a weak cough, but it was too painful.

"Do you want me to stick this tube back in your throat?" she insisted.

"I really don't care," Lad replied. "Just don't make me cough."

Three days later, Lad was released and back in control. It would not take him long to get back in the swing of things.

Chapter 18

July 29, 1999

It was Thursday, July 29, 1999. Lad was at the Experimental Aircraft Association's 47th annual Air Venture in Oshkosh, Wisconsin, his 19th year to perform at the annual gathering of aviation enthusiasts, the largest of its kind in the world. 800,000 people attended, making the airport's control tower the busiest in the world during the event.

Some of the WWII enthusiasts lined the flight line at Wittman Regional Airport just to see the Vought F4U Corsair. It had the longest production run of any piston-engine fighter in U.S. history and was one of WWII's greatest fighter planes. It could outfight, outclimb and outrun any propeller-driven enemy aircraft.

The pilot sat in a large cockpit over the wing trailing edge. The view straight forward over the engine cowling was poor, even more so than common in single-seat fighters of the day. View to the sides was rea-

sonable, although the cockpit canopy was heavily framed. No concessions were made to rearward view, the aft of the cockpit being faired into a gently sloping fuselage decking. The tail planes and fins had rounded tips, and the control surfaces were fabric covered.

Armament consisted of one .50 gun in each wing, and a .50 and a .30 in the engine cowl decking. There was also room for 20 small anti-aircraft bombs, stored in the wings....[26]

World War II pilots did it all without the benefit of an ejection seat.

Not one person standing on the flight line that day could have imagined what this aircraft meant to Lad. In his eyes this plane was a symbol of the many heroes who stepped inside the cockpit and the technology of that era. It stood for a horrific war and the heroes who fought for freedom in that plane. He polished it and maintained every inch of it.

All eyes were on Lad as he walked toward the beautiful blue Corsair and climbed into the cockpit. At age 56, he had four flight certificates allowing him to fly airline transports, helicopters, gliders, and single and multi-engine airplanes. To that point, Lad had accumulated over 8,000 flight hours in almost 100 different aircraft, including military turbojets. He still has the original flight manuals for almost every World War II, Korean and Vietnam-era aircraft he has ever flown.

That was Lad's life until July 29, 1999 at 2:30 in the afternoon. He was about to take off at the busiest airport in the world because of this event.

It may have been a very distracting time for the Air Boss because he knew Lad's program, a four-plane tandem takeoff: two Bearcats followed by two Corsairs.

Lad was in the #3 spot. Because of the Corsair's high nose and aft-placed cockpit, he could not see in front of him while taxiing, but he knew the program, just as Stevie Wonder was sure of which keys to play. And he also trusted that the Air Boss would be his eyes from the moment he started his takeoff roll until he rotated the tail up. This event accumulated 12,000 or more airplanes, so Lad knew the Air Boss had to be qualified.

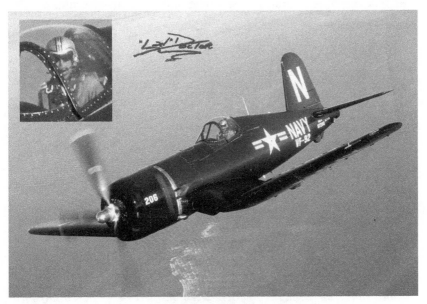

Lad flying the Corsair over the Houston ship channel in September of 1996.
The Corsair was on the back cover of GHOSTS-1998.
©PhilipMakanna/GHOSTS

It wasn't all about the beautiful blue airplane he had climbed into—there was a Vietnam Veteran in that plane. Over the years Lad had garnered international respect in every area of aviation and his aeronautical ability, knowledge and judgement were highly sought-after and respected. He had piloted an A-5 Vigilante during the Vietnam War. He had served as the Federal Aviation Administration Designee for Pylon Racing. He was Chairman of the AT-6 Racing Association, an AT-6 check pilot, and had helped create FAA guidelines to keep wannabe race pilots and spectators safe. He was involved in the National Air Races, he was Chief Pilot and Director of Cavanaugh's Flight Museum, and he even choreographed flight patterns. He helped organize the first Airshow at Alliance Airfield in Fort Worth, Texas. Colonel Mario Cafiero knew the hundreds of children

Lad piloted over Plant 42 in Palmdale, California, were in great hands. On this day, for a few brief minutes, Lad would need to trust someone else to be the expert. Someone else would have to be his eyes until he could see over the nose of the plane.

He pushed the throttle full forward to begin his takeoff roll.

The spectators could see what Lad could not see, and most importantly, the Air Boss could see what Lad could not see.

Witnesses that day said:

"According to eyewitness reports, the northbound Corsair hit the Bearcat, one of two airplanes that had come to a stop on the edge of the runway."[27]

Another witness said:

"Two of them had stopped for whatever reason, I don't know why. The Corsairs were taking off and one of them just plowed right into the Bearcat," Lawson said. "I can't understand why they (the Corsairs) were cleared with a crosswind when there are two planes on the runway."[28]

Another said:

"When I saw it I couldn't understand why the Bearcat was going so slow, it didn't make sense," said Joe Neff, a pilot from Indianapolis.[29]

And a very telling eyewitness, Craig Yancy said, "I was standing under their controls (Airboss) and could hear every conversation with the pilots. They never warned Lad to hold off."

The four pilots had flown this program numerous times. At this time the Oshkosh tower turned the control of Wittman Airfield over to the Air Boss. The Air Boss' duty was to report any and all information critical to the pilots' safety and the safety of others. It wasn't until Lad could obtain the speed needed to raise the tail that he could see the horrific sight right in front of him.

Lad and Jim Reed assumed that the two Bearcats, one flown by Howard Pardue and the other by Tom Wood, had already taken off.

"At the show, we were flying a formation with two Bearcats in front of us," said Lad. "Mr. Pardue had a wingman just as I did. Once we took off we would have separated ourselves to be in formation, but in trail with a whole lot of planes behind. I didn't know there was going to be an accident until the tail came up and there were two airplanes. My speed was at a point that I tried to make a turn and rotate the right wing down, left wing up, to go between the two aircraft and I clearly went by the second Bearcat and to this day, in my mind's eye picture, I looked over and will swear I saw Howard in the cockpit and I was above him and I thought I made it.

"I felt a little bump in the fuselage of the Corsair, in my lower right quadrant, a little aft of where I was sitting. It all happened in a flash. The nose was down and the engine, with the propeller turning, running away from me in a long arching left-hand turn, coming to rest in the dirt on the left side of the runway," said Lad.

At the point of impact, the Corsair clipped the right wing off the Bearcat, which pointed up at a 45-degree angle before coming to rest facing the opposite direction.

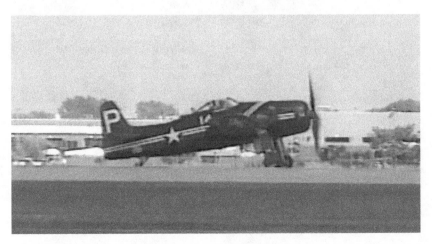

Bearcat. *Courtesy of WBAY-TV*

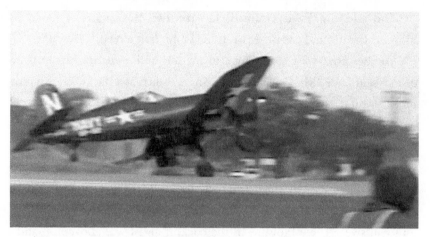

At the point of impact, the Corsair clipped the right wing off the Bearcat, which pointed up at a 45 degree angle before coming to rest facing the opposite direction.
Courtesy of WBAY-TV

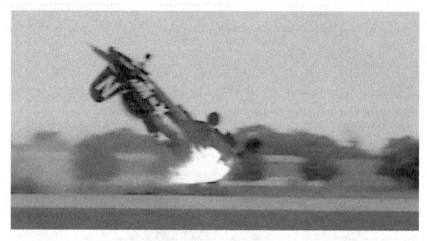

"The Corsair spun off to the west side of the runway and began cartwheeling into the grass, where it lay burning until emergency crews arrived," said John Lawson, of Louisville, Kentucky, who witnessed the crash.
Courtesy of WBAY-TV

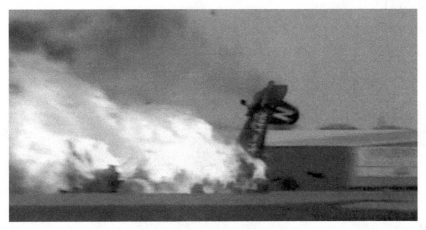

Courtesy of WBAY-TV

"The Corsair spun off to the west side of the runway and began cartwheeling into the grass, where it lay burning until emergency crews arrived," said John Lawson, of Louisville, Kentucky, who witnessed the crash.

The broken plane lay scattered in pieces, blazing horrifically.

"The plane breaks into three main parts," said Lad. "The engine and the tail broke away. Everything in between was one part. But I wasn't in the center section. The back of my seat was attached to the bulkhead, which I was strapped too. The seat cushion was cantilevered into the cockpit. I was actually attached to the monocoque. The plane broke apart right at that bulkhead. The fire and everything forward of the bulkhead was away from me. The whole tail end of the airplane went somewhere else with me hanging out the front of it. The seat was firmly bolted into the back part of the plane. The crash crew assumed that I was sitting in the cockpit."

Fortunately, one spectator did not hale to the loud broadcasts demanding that everyone Stay out of the way.

"There was a guy in the audience who came to my rescue," said Lad. "I don't have his name. I was told that he was a trained NASCAR paramedic whose natural instinct was to run toward the wreckage as it was taking place. He cut me loose and pulled me from the wreckage to a safe location within seconds."

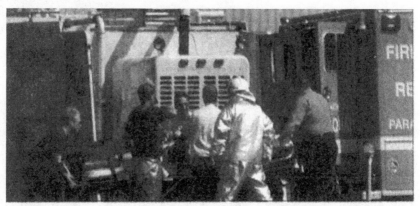

LAIRD DOCTOR is loaded into an emergency vehicle after a plane crash at the EAA AirVenture grounds Thursday afternoon.

Front page news. *Courtesy of Oshkosh Northwestern*

"The National Transportation Safety Board (NTS) guys said there wasn't one part of the airplane that wasn't damaged. It blew up and broke apart." Later, as proof of the sickening violence of the crash, airplane parts were found scattered everywhere.

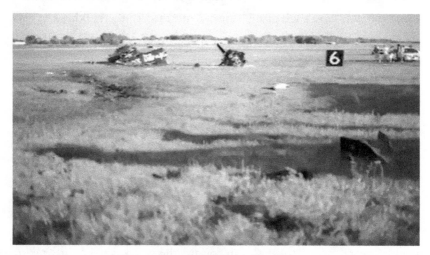

The wreckage. *Compliments of Laird Doctor*

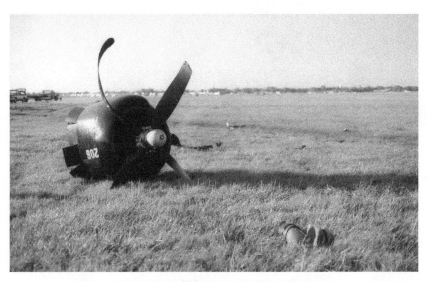

The wreckage. *Compliments of Laird Doctor*

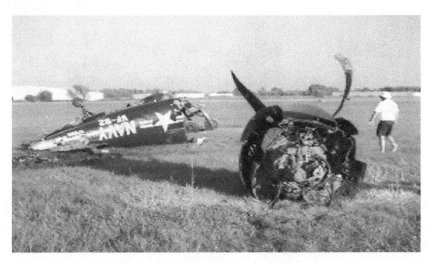

The wreckage. *Compliments of Laird Doctor*

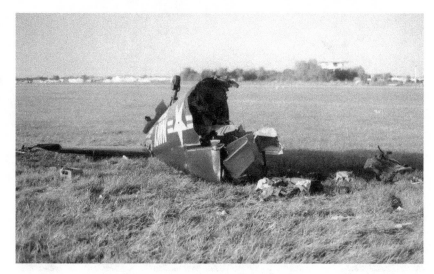

Compliments of Laird Doctor

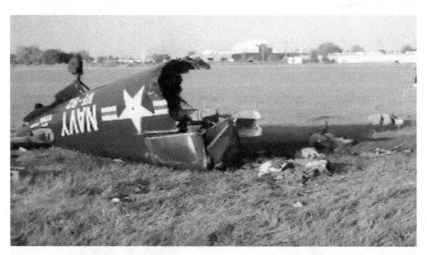

Compliments of Laird Doctor

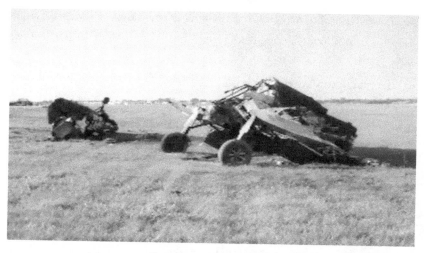

Compliments of Laird Doctor

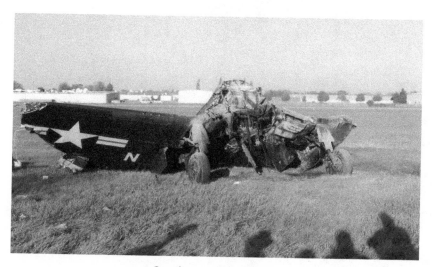

Compliments of Laird Doctor

"Do you know where Katie is?" asked Lauren Rambo. "There has been an accident."

At that time, Katie and her now ex-husband worked for the same company, and she was at his desk when he received the call.

Lauren Rambo was Jim Cavanaugh's executive assistant and Katie's friend. From where she sat, Katie could hear the urgency in her friend's voice.

"Do you know where Katie is?"

Katie grabbed the phone.

"Jim Cavanaugh's private jet has left Oshkosh," Lauren said. "It will be in Addison and available to take you and Linda to Oshkosh."

Katie could not make it to the airport in time, so the pilot returned the next morning and flew her and Lauren to Oshkosh.

"I could not have made it through those first couple of days without Lauren," remembered Katie.

Reporters hovered as they tried to make sense of it all. Lad was front page news.

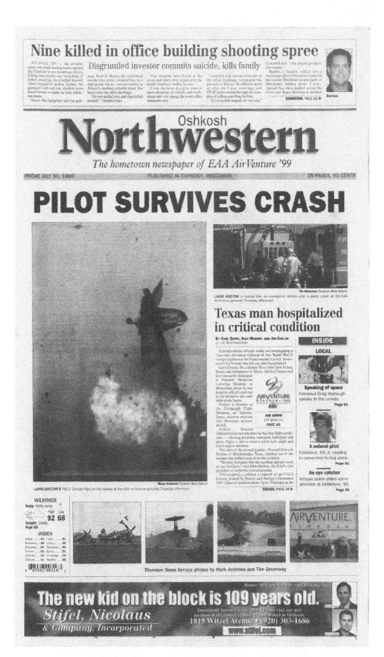

Oshkosh Northwestern, "Pilot Survives Crash."
Courtesy of Oshkosh Northwestern

Chapter 19

The Powerful White

Doctors would not know the extent of Lad's injuries for several months, but it was apparent there had been substantial damage to his spine. He had a million questions, but was unable to speak due to the respirator and other tubes in his mouth.

> *Federal aviation officials today are investigating a Thursday afternoon collision of two World War II vintage airplanes at the Experimental Aircraft Association's Air Venture that left one pilot hospitalized.*
>
> *Laird Doctor, 56, a former Navy pilot from Frisco, Texas was transported to Mercy Medical Center and later moved by helicopter to Froedtert Memorial Lutheran Hospital* [30]

The accident, and more importantly, Lad, would be the scuttlebutt across the globe. Friends, family, co-workers, and fellow aviation enthusiasts prayed.

The pilot of the second airplane, Howard Edwards Pardue of Breckenridge, Texas, climbed out of the airplane and walked away from the accident.[31]

The EAA's vice president of corporate communication said, "We were fortunate that the accident did not result in any fatalities."

The accident, a collision at takeoff of an F4U-1 Corsair piloted by Doctor and Pardue's Grumman F8F-1 Bearcat occurred...

According to eyewitness reports, the northbound Corsair hit the Bearcat, one of two airplanes that had come to a stop on the edge of the runway.

Groups of warbirds owners huddled on the airport grounds near the three remaining Corsairs at the show, consoling each other and discussing the accident. As a group they declined to talk to the press, referring questions to the EAA's warbirds headquarters.

One witness said the professionalism and training of the airshow pilots made the accident especially disturbing.

"It was a shock," said the man, who asked to remain anonymous. "It was 'open mouth, what the hell happened' shock. This is the last place any of us would expect this."

"When I saw it I couldn't understand why the Bearcat was going so slow, it didn't make sense," said Joe Neff, a pilot from Indianapolis.[32]

Lad's fears were too vast to comprehend. The accident left him paralyzed from the neck down, with limited movement in his neck due to significant damage to his spinal cord, not to mention that Lad was still healing from open heart surgery.

"And my memory is not too clear for about six months after the accident," said Lad. He can remember things transpiring around him, namely involving family and medical staff. "I can remember those kinds of things, but I can't put them together in any time continuum or in any geographical place. I don't know if it took place in the emergency room at Oshkosh or in Milwaukee, or in the hospital in Dallas or at the hospital in Denver. I just remember *things* happening, but for the most part, it is a mystery to me."

After being rushed to a Milwaukee hospital in critical condition, Lad's condition was upgraded to critical but stable by late Friday night. From there, Lad was transferred to Froedtert Memorial Lutheran Hospital, also in Milwaukee.

"It's a miracle that you did not catch on fire," said the doctor. "Or break your arms or legs because of the ferocious way that you were thrown around."

Those would not be the only miracles. Somewhere within the first three months of the accident Lad would experience something so brilliant and magnificent that words could never fully capture its true glory.

"I can't tell you where or when," said Lad. "But I know it was 100% real."

As Lad lay in bed, fully conscience and fully awake, an intense "white" appeared. "The *strength* of the sublime *'white'* was very significant," said Lad. "It was *white*. It wasn't a dream or a hallucination. It was real. Then three angels with gossamer wings hovered over me. One was at the foot of my bed and one on each side of me. I often wonder if a fourth angel could have been behind me since there seemed to be one on each side. The angels were *there*. I knew instinctively they were protecting me and it gave me great strength. At that instant, a very clear voice said, 'When the angels return, they'll bring you home.'

"I'm not done yet. I didn't turn to the LORD," said Lad. "He took hold of me."

Shortly thereafter, Lad struggled to understand a vision that would not stop. Why was it constantly racing through his thoughts? The vision would not let go. It devoured his mental state and it meant absolutely nothing to him.

Lad can't imagine how he could have possibly communicated with Linda, but he did. He had to make sense of it all, maybe relaying the message to someone would clear his thoughts.

Linda must have read his lips, which that too is a miracle with the tubes in the way.

"A thought keeps racing through my mind," He told her. "Something about green pastures and water. It doesn't make any sense."

"That is the 23rd Psalm," Linda replied.

Other than traditional Jewish celebrations, Lad knew very little to nothing about the teachings in the Bible and had no recollection of ever hearing or reading the 23rd Psalm.

"I don't recall having ever read the Bible prior to the accident," he said.

Linda continued,

"The LORD is my shepherd; I shall not be in want
He maketh me lie down in green pastures, he leads me beside quiet
    waters,
He restores my soul.
He guides me in paths of righteousness
For his name's sake.
Even though I walk through the valley of the shadow of death
I will fear no evil
For you are with me
Your rod and your staff they comfort me.
You prepare a table before me in the presence of my enemies.
You anoint my head with oil; my cup overflows
Surely goodness and love will follow me all the days of my life
And I will dwell in the house of the LORD forever."

"I never could retain information instantaneously," said Lad. "Yet, after hearing Linda recite the Psalm for the first and only time, I remembered it verbatim."

At this point, Lad could have never fathomed the mental toil of medical tests and problems that lay ahead for him. While inside the small, confined quarters of the loud, enclosed MRI chamber, he repeated,

"The Lord is my shepherd; I shall not be in want."

Lad had been given a means to cope. No one sat by his bed making suggestions. The Psalm came to him. And it would be the 23rd Psalm that would get Lad through horrific anxiety and medical tests too numerous to grasp.

"The Lord is my shepherd."

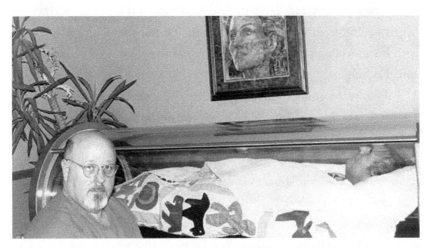

Infusing oxygen to the damaged area using the Hyperbaric Chamber
for one hour, three times a day for one year.
Compliments of Laird Doctor

The visions continued. Lad saw himself crawling on the ground next to a large crowd trying to touch Jesus.

"Jesus wore a white robe," said Lad. "With a gold sash, and there was a two-inch gold trim around the bottom of his robe. I know because I was tugging at the bottom of it trying to get his attention."

He turned and looked, but never lowered his gaze. Again, Lad tugged and this time Jesus saw him.

"Jesus reached down towards me," said Lad. "When he touched my head, I could feel all my pain drain out from the top of my head all the way down my body, and out through my feet. And the vision stopped there."

A Jew witnessed Jesus.

Lad, a man nurtured in the Jewish faith, who never questioned his upbringing, witnessed Jesus. Lad never had a second thought of who Jesus was or why he was giving Lad comfort. Lad's life was unfolding before him. Intense anxiety and the fear of never moving again overwhelmed him.

The hospital room was full of beeping machines, tubes and wires everywhere, day in and day out. And to trouble his thoughts further, be began feeling a sense of regret and guilt for not spending quality time with his mother and father before their passing. Lad wasn't reaching for spiritual help.

"What was I going to do?" Lad asked. "Worse even, what could I do? I had a dream. I was sitting in a wheelchair, in the aisle of a church in San Antonio, Texas. From my chair, I looked up and witnessed Jesus himself on the cross in Jerusalem. Jesus was reaching down to me with his right hand. I often thought about that dream and it makes no anatomical sense that Jesus could reach down."

Sometime later, after immersing himself in the Bible, he would learn that Jesus had suffered thrashing and beatings that peeled the skin off of his body until he was unrecognizable by even those who loved him.

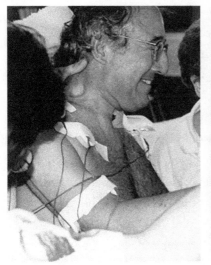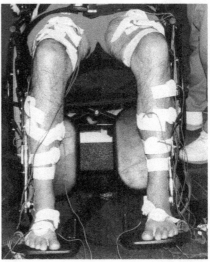

Electrodes and exercise.
Compliments of Laird Doctor

For God sent not his Son into the world to condemn the world; but that the world through him might be saved.

But he that doeth truth cometh to the light, that his deeds may be made manifest, that they are wrought in GOD.

-John 3:16 KJV

That *light* . . . .

Lad couldn't stop the ongoing regrets and guilt of missing an opportunity to spend more time with his parents. Then God gave Lad freedom from regret and guilt in what would be his final vision.

"There were numerous escalators and flights of stairs everywhere I turned," said Lad. "Those walking the stairs were descending and those being lifted on the escalators were ascending."

Lad's eyes followed the escalators to the top, and there stood Jesus.

Lad had been living with agonizing guilt for not being the son he felt he should have been during his mother and father's final days. It was then that God freed Lad of all stress connected to his parents.

"As those escalators continued upward," said Lad. "My mother and father were standing together, looking down on me and smiling, 'We're all right.'"

"I was such an independent cuss," said Lad. "If I had the use of my arms, I would be at the gym every day making sure that my upper body was muscular. If I had any control, I would have never turned to the Lord. I would have never listened. I would have continued to think that I was in control. The Lord had to get me into a position where I was unable to look to myself for anything. God knew that the only way that he was going to get me to understand that I can't do it without him was to prove it. So, you better come this way. The Lord was telling me something for sure."

Lad had more than 14 surgeries to repair the extensive damage the crash had done to his body.

"It took a long time to physically overcome the various surgeries," remembered Lad. "But it took even longer to overcome the mental side effects to such a life-altering situation. I would not have lived this long if it had not been for Michael and Susy Jouett," referring to Jouett Respiratory Therapy Associates in Lewisville, Texas.

"DRI stands for Dallas Rehabilitation Institute," explained Michael Jouett. "DRI 'protocol' for cervical (high) spinal cord injury (SCI) rehabilitation. While it was open, DRI had the most advanced program for SCI rehabilitation in the United States. The initial, pioneering work in the program's development was carried out by two respiratory therapists, David Moseley and Malcolm May. Their work was carried out with the support and collaboration of Dr. George Wharton, one of the foremost spinal surgeons in Dallas at that time. Later, medical direction for the program was assumed by a pulmonologist, Dr. Joseph Viroslav, who advanced the program and who remains one of the leading pulmonary experts in cervical SCI rehabilitation.

"The assisted cough technique was one of the break-through treatments developed by this group. The basic technique involved training the patient to 'cough' with assistance from a respiratory therapist. Cervical SCI involves paralysis of the abdominal muscles, the major muscle group employed in the natural cough. The diaphragm, the major muscle of inspiration, is also partly or wholly paralyzed, depending on the level of the spinal injury. The respiratory therapist assists the patient to cough by first using a breathing machine or a resuscitation bag to give the patient a deep breath. Then, cuing the patient to cough, he/she sharply compresses the abdomen, forcing air up and out and expelling accumulated secretions. This technique, when effectively applied, eliminates the need for deep tracheal suctioning with the associated tracheal and carinal injury. It is also much more effective than tracheal suctioning in that it moves secretions up and out that are well beyond the reach of a suction catheter."

Lad fears others will never benefit from this process once Michael Jouett retires. "They are the only company that uses this technique in extreme respiratory needs," said Lad. "Probably in the world I guess."

The first operation on Lad's neck was at Zale Lipshy at UT Southwestern in Dallas. Miraculously, the respiratory technician on call that night, and who also trained at DRI, administered the same techniques that Michael's company practices.

"Usually, when a trached patient coughs or chokes," said Lad, "a flexible tube is attached on the trach, which is connected to a machine that pulls secretions out of the lungs. This tube creates yet another agitation. Because it is a foreign substance, the body's defense mechanism produces increased secretion. So, the procedure of extracting the secretion makes more secretion, and is a vicious circle, a never-ending cycle. Every time I coughed—'Oh, here comes the suctioning'—because I no longer have the muscles needed to create an effective cough."

During Lad's stay, another angel of sorts walked into his room.

"What were the odds?" Lad asked. He might not have stood a chance if not for this man. Few respiratory technicians understood the special DRI techniques.

Miraculously, Eric Johnston did.

"Every night, Eric helped me cough naturally using the DRI techniques," said Lad. "He created the same effect as a cough by squeezing and constricting my body. It was no longer in my chest so he could suction from my throat, without equipment and without that tube in my chest. What are the odds that out of all the hospitals in the area, and the different areas within the hospital, that the one guy trained at DRI would not only be at the same hospital, but on the night shift? The stars and planets have to be aligned for this to take place. And that is just one little part of all the things that took place that kept me alive. That got me to this point. It has to make a believer out of you. It has to. There is just no other logical answer. It's just too complex for all these things to align themselves. I don't believe that I would have ever left the hospital if it had not been for Eric Johnston."

§

Then there was the horrific trial regarding the accident.

"The deposition and trial was quite lengthy and really quite strenuous on me," remembered Lad. "Not mentally, physically. Even now, my endurance is not like a normal person. I get tired pretty easily. At that time, boy, I didn't go anywhere, and I didn't do anything, and everything was a real struggle. It still is darn inconvenient to go places, but at least I can go. He smiles. And do things."

§

Lad was on his way for rehab at a well-known institute in Denver, Colorado.

"Rehab to me meant the doctors and staff would make sure that every effort would be made to see that any area of hope would be tested, exercised and strengthened," said Lad. "I knew that the first year of recovery was the most important and I was eager to get started. Turned out, it wasn't rehabilitation as advertised, it was adaptation. Their practice of rehabilitation consisted of being lined up along the wall with other quadriplegics next to the nurse's station.

"Let's get busy. Let's work to regain every possible body function available. Don't stick me next to a wall and forget about me. This is a thrill. Can I go back to my room and watch television? While there, I was sick and just existing."

During Lad's time at the institute, he was treated for pulmonary problems and they would not take him off the ventilator. His lung had atelectasis.

"Atelectasis refers to partial collapse of lung units and is a particular problem to patients on ventilators who are not routinely treated with deep breathing assistance/therapy," said Michael Jouett. "Atelectasis quickly forms in gravity-dependent lung regions, leading to pneumonia and reductions in blood oxygen levels. Deep breathing therapy is administered by briefly taking the patient off the ventilator and administering deep breaths at volumes up to the patient's inspiratory capacity. Assisted cough techniques are also best applied in conjunction with deep breath therapy."

The left side of Lad's diaphragm is paralyzed, which means the right side must do the work for both sides. The health care professionals at the institute concluded that, on a good day, Lad might get relief from the ventilator for a couple of hours, but he'd never be totally weaned.

"My lung X-rays were white-ish which meant that there wasn't any air in my lung," Lad explained. Muscle is needed in order to take a deep breath. Quadriplegics lack that muscle and the ventilator makes it worse."

Anxiety attacks consumed Lad after just 40 minutes of being off the ventilator. Lad feared he would die without it. Breathing was no longer a natural occurrence for him. He had to walk himself through the action of breathing.

"I've gotta inhale, I've gotta exhale. Inhale, exhale. And that in itself produces anxiety," said Lad. "I can't even explain my mental state. I was coming undone. About 45 minutes into it, 'I need a vent, I need a vent, I need a vent.' I was bonkers—out of my mind—'I need a vent, I need a vent. Help me. I'm dying here. I'm suffocating. I'm dying.'"

Lad was scared for his life. He was placed back on the ventilator and the staff declared, "We can't get him weaned."

Chapter 20

Damn

Linda flew Eric to Denver.

After Eric and the staff met, Eric looked at the equipment attached to Lad and said, "Jiminy Christmas. It's obvious what is wrong. You are introducing carbon dioxide into his cycle of breathing and now his body wants to maintain that high level of CO_2."

Grudgingly, the pulmonary team allowed Eric to work on Lad.

"Sure... I will do whatever he wants for a week," mimicked Lad. "What the hell. Go ahead take your shot."

Eric added a humidifier and had Lad weaned in two days.

Before he left, Eric said, "Lad, don't worry about what they say, you are weaned. At 4:00 a.m., Friday morning, before I return to Texas and before they take X-rays, I will do a full treatment on you. I know you will be okay. Try not to be anxious."

Following Eric's treatment, the pulmonologist placed Lad's X-ray next to the window.

"My lungs were clear from top to bottom," Lad remembered. "Not a white mark anywhere."

"Damn," the doctor said.

"Isn't that something?" Lad questioned. "'Damn' was his comment. I remember it so clearly. I was sitting right there. Looks at it, my lungs are perfect. It proved this procedure can clear me up."

But now Eric was gone and Lad watched in horror as they began reattaching all the equipment.

More than once, friends and colleagues had asked Lad to keep an eye on their business partners, the safety of their aircraft and the safety of those who wanted to fly, but now someone needed to keep an eye out for Lad. Within two days after Eric Johnston left, Lad's lungs were full and he was back on the machine.

"If you take Lad out of here, you're going to kill him," the staff declared.

After only three months of the nine-month rehabilitation program, Lad left Denver disappointed.

Lad, Linda and Eric, who Linda had now hired full time, were on their way to Florida.

§

The door flew open and there stood an Angel. They had just settled into their hotel room when Lane Hubbard stopped by with lunch.

Lad had been on a feeding tube for close to six months.

"I will never forget it," remembered Lad. "Lane brought me a Subway sandwich. Oh my gosh, the taste of that thing was magnificent. It was amazing. I could taste everything that was in that sandwich. The lettuce. Ooooh, the lettuce was so good. The tomato, ooooh the tomato was so good. The bread is so good and the sauce, whatever it is, ahhhh. The flavors were so pungent. And I could distinctly taste every flavor in that sandwich. Oh my gosh, what a treat that was."

> 3 aug '99
>
> Dear Lad,
> I'm hoping and praying to God every day and night for your recovery!! You know I've been there!" So I can imagine how you feel.
> God took care of me, Lad, and I'm continually asking him to take care of you! He will!!
> — Love to you, Lynda Katie. Charlie Bond

Dear Lad, Charlie Bond. *Compliments of Laird Doctor*

"Is there anything else you can think of that you want?" Lane asked.

"Pizza!" Lad said. "I want a piece of pizza."

"I'll bring you a pizza," Lane said.

"Can I have another Subway?" asked Lad.

"I was so preoccupied," remembered Lad. "Where are we going? Let me see the menu. I was just talking away. I felt almost human, except in really bad shape."

But his life was very different now. While at the restaurant, Eric and Lad had to excuse themselves from the dining table and find a place to clear Lad's lungs.

CONFEDERATE AIR FORCE, INC.

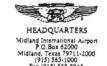

HEADQUARTERS
Midland International Airport
P.O. Box 62000
Midland, Texas 79711-2000
(915) 563-1000
Fax (915) 563-8046

FAX TRANSMITTAL SHEET

TO: Lad Doctor   ATTN: NICU

FAX NUMBER: 414 259 1244

FROM: Bob Rice

FAX NUMBER: 915-563-8046

DATE: 3 AUG 99

NO. OF PAGES INCLUDING COVER: 1

IF YOU DO NOT RECEIVE ALL THE PAGES, PLEASE CALL 915-563-1000.

Lad — all of your friends in the CAF, and there are a bunch of us, want you to know that we're thinking about you and Linda. We are told that you are receiving the best care possible and are able to take comfort in knowing this. However, we need you back in our "RANKS" just as fast as you can get here!
  Take good care of yourself, get some rest and know that all you have to do is call on us if and when we can assist you and your family in any way.

Warmest Regards,
Bob & Friends

Compliments of Laird Doctor

Additional surgeries would require the trach, and the weaning process would repeat itself. But the get-well cards, letters and emails came from around the world.

Lad needed 24-hour care: Nurses, caregivers, medications, appliances, cooks, home modifications, transportation, and more. It was all worth it because he did not want to spend the rest of his life in a rest home staring at a television set. Lad's life, however, would be costly to sustain.

"It takes A LOT, A LOT of money to keep me going," said Lad. "And not everyone with my level of injury has workman's compensation. I would have been a statistic and dead in seven years had it not been for workman's compensation. I was able to covert my home to quadriplegic friendly."

Lad testified, in explicit detail, concerning the physical pain and mental suffering that he has experienced. He described the indignity he feels as a result of his condition and his constant need for assistance in performing the most basic of human functions. Lad related his feelings of depression when he discovered that, despite every effort at rehabilitation, he would never walk again and would always need a ventilator to breathe. Lad also noted that during one particular treatment, when a tube was inserted into his throat, he gagged, his jaw cracked, and he experienced severe discomfort. Lad explained that suctioning performed on him during treatment is very uncomfortable and that breathing through a ventilator is also very uncomfortable. When his blood pressure is elevated, Lad experiences headaches and painful tightening of his neck.

Lad is fearful that his ventilator may stop working or that he will be dropped when being transferred or moved. Lad is also fearful that he may be injured by someone attempting to assist.

The doctors also presented extensive evidence concerning Lad's hospitalization, and the pain and suffering that he has experienced during those hospitalizations. Immediately after the collision, Lad was taken to a local medical center and then transferred to a spinal cord injury unit at another hospital, where he stayed for one week. While there, he was placed on a ventilator and fed through a stomach tube. Linda testified that Lad was terrified. Lad was then transferred to another hospital for continued spinal cord care, and remained at that hospital for another month. There, Lad underwent decompression surgery to stabilize his neck, during which pins were inserted into his neck to hold it in place. These metal pins cause Lad pain. While at this medical center, Lad could not communicate with anyone, make any sound, or press a call button to summon the assistance of the nurses. Lad could not move his head, but he did experience discomfort in his head, and was medicated for that discomfort. Lad also was strapped to a board to completely immobilize him.

Lad was then transferred to another care facility for rehabilitation, where he remained for another two months. There, Lad suffered from numerous medical conditions and complications, including pneumonia, respiratory problems, infections, hypertension, and anemia.[33]

Every two weeks, Lad sees a psychologist, who is also wheelchair-bound and with whom he has become a genuine friend. Lad feels at this point in his treatment that they help each other.

"I should charge him," Lad declares, laughing.

"Wheelchairs handle really well if you can use your hands," said Lad. "You have the ability to control the speed, which is important. With the sip and puff method, I have to ramp up to go fast and ramp down to go slow or the chair stops all together. The sip and puff method doesn't work as well. But if God had left me with any of those capabilities, I would have never listened."

Michael Jouett started a Bible study class that meets weekly at Lad's home, which has enforced his trust in God amid trying times such as struggles with medical staff who did not and do not understand the simple appliances needed to sustain him.

"I can't attach the footrest back onto your wheelchair," said the nurse.

Though Lad is unable to look down or turn his head, he walked the nurse through the steps on how to reattach it.

"There is a yellow line on the chair," Lad explained to the nurse. "And a yellow arrow on the footrest. Put the footrest in the hole, then line it up with the yellow arrow."

To keep himself alive, Lad must learn as much as possible about every procedure the medical staff must perform so that when a caretaker doesn't understand, or unknowingly is in the act of making a costly mistake, he can speak up.

Lad believes he is here today to accomplish God's plans. On December 9, 1999, Lad received an email from Craig Yancey, a witness to the accident, affirming this:

> *"Dear Mr. Doctor, I am glad that the news on the website implies that you are doing somewhat better. I have and do pray for you and your family since this accident. I witnessed it happen and watched it unfold from directly across the taxiway from it. I, along with hundreds of people around me, stopped and said a prayer for you after the incident. I don't know exactly what you are going through, but it isn't easy, I'm sure of that. I want to thank you for the effort that you and the people you flew with, to share with us, your love of aviation. I love the warbirds for their strength and power that they represent, not for the power to destroy but their power to protect. Keep working and improve something each day, you will be back at home soon. Hang in there, and say a prayer for yourself, it's allowed. A long lost fellow Texan, Craig Yancey."*

And on May 11, 2017, Craig Yancey followed up with a letter to the author:

> *...I still think about it quite frequently.*
>
> *I spent 12 years working as a Firefighter/Paramedic on the E.R.T. (Emergency Response Team), at the "Sun-n-Fun Fly In" in Lakeland, Florida (that's the southern version of Oshkosh or Air Venture.)*
>
> *So with my background in A.R.F.F. (Aircraft Rescue Fire Fighting), and as a pilot myself, I was a member of the ERT Entry Team known as "The Hammerheads" where we were responsible to stabilize the*

scene, extinguish fires, and extricate pilots and passengers from aircraft involved in any type of incident.

In other words, I feel that I have a little professional background to base my opinions on.

During those years, I witnessed and participated in many aircraft incidents and crashes, and had hands-on experience with many different levels of events.

Lad's is still the worst accident that I've seen, and to have it unfold right before me, and to be feeling so helpless to prevent it..., that still haunts me.

...I was completely unaware of the legal situation that he became embroiled in.

...It is so fantastic to see Lad doing "well," considering that the last time I saw him (which was 20 minutes after the accident when they were removing him from the scene), I knew in my heart that he was deceased.

I really didn't think that a human could have lived through that violent of an accident, that fire, and what seemed to me to be a long extrication time. God is Good, All the time!

From what I saw and read online, Lad was given a raw deal by the court system. There is no way that he was 50% responsible for the crash!

Justice is not a part of our legal system.

In my opinion, the jury should have been made up of people who actually witnessed the crash.

Since I was standing beneath a speaker system that was broadcasting live the radio communications of the Air Boss with the aircraft, I firmly believe that the Air Boss and his staff were the leading cause for that accident.

They have the only "link" to the pilots via radio, and they must always stay vigilant to the fact that those pilots rely on them to be their eyes while they are in the beginning stage of their takeoff runs.

There were NO warnings given by the Air Boss, to any aircraft (especially those aircraft who were in the staging area and preparing to depart), that there was any type of situation with the first wave of aircraft that had just "launched," and that the remaining aircraft should "hold short" or to abort their takeoff.

The pilots of that type of aircraft cannot see the runway directly in front of them, UNTIL they obtain the speed sufficient to raise their tails. Therefore, the Air Boss and his staff are to focus their undivided attention on the task of safely launching each of the aircraft.

Sorry to have vented, but watching those videos caused my old feelings to resurface and it really angers me to know that the majority of the blame for this accident was somehow shifted to Lad. I'm sure that Lad does accept a part of the responsibility for the accident, since he was the Pilot In Command (PIC), but that portion should not be deemed so large.

When you communicate with Lad, please let him know that there are still people who think about him, and that they all wish him well!

Best Regards,
W. Craig Yancey
Yancey Aviation, LLC

"There was enough blame to go around," said Lad. Laird Ashley Doctor now has the fight of his life. His fears are too many to comprehend.

"The nurses lifted me out of bed at 1:00 in the afternoon," remembered Lad. "Then to the wheel and mat for roughly four hours of exercise followed by dinner and a gazillion pills."

Sometime after the accident, Lad recalled the day he was riding his bicycle and had overstepped his authority when he declared, "YOU… CAN'T…MAKE…IT…TOUGH…ENOUGH."

"I realized God could make it tough enough," said Lad. "And then some." The accident has left him paralyzed from the neck down, with limited movement in his neck due to significant damage to his spinal cord. He is a very high-level quadriplegic. His vertebrae are crushed from #2 to #4. Had he broken one more vertebra, he would not have survived. His entire neck from cervical #2 to #7, are fused together. His neck doesn't curve and has a limited forward and backward movement. All the nerves below #2 are dead. The cervical spine, the topmost portion of the spine, consists of seven vertebrae (C1-C7), each with a pair of nerves on each side to serve various functions in the upper body. In principle, with a complete injury of the cervical spine, all bodily functions served by these nerves from the thoracic and lumbar spine are also affected.

Lad can breathe on his own during the day, but at night he is on noninvasive ventilation for safety. He cannot produce an effective cough and has no bowel or bladder control. Because his abdominal muscles are paralyzed, he is unable to speak loudly and sometimes fragments sentences so he can take a breath.

Lad uses a powered wheelchair controlled with a "sip–puff" device that requires a lot of skill to operate. He needs 24-hour-a-day personal care. Because Lad can't stand up, squirm or cross his legs to increase blood flow, every 30 minutes a nurse must lean the back of his wheel chair backwards for 90 seconds. This takes the pressure off his bottom and improves circulation. His body senses the change in movement causing his hands to spasm. He can't perform any normal function without help.

Life in a wheelchair sometimes causes his neck to ache, and in order to keep his kidneys from failing, he must drink three liters of water a day.

"Pressure sores and wounds are unfortunately more common in spinal cord injury patients," said Michael Jouett. "Due to the loss of sensation, an individual will not realize a wound is developing, and it may become somewhat advanced before a caregiver spots it. If any of the involved tissue has died, it will be very difficult for the wound to heal on its own. After a round of care from a wound specialist, some wounds just have to be surgically resected."

§

Instead of Lad's two-wheeler (motorcycle), he now drives a 400-pound four-wheeler. "Just trying to live a normal life with a normal routine is maybe the biggest challenge I see Lad face," says Milo Ruch, a close friend and former employee. "His disability requires a lot of 'body maintenance' as Lad calls it, just for him to be up and about. Whereas most people could be up, dressed, eat and out the door in five or ten minutes, the whole process for Lad takes two to three hours, even when things go right. It goes without saying that a lot of patience is required for that kind of a daily routine."

Terry the Torch and Lad had lost contact for a few years. "Something was telling me to find Laddie," said Terry. "While in Paso Robles, California, there was a plaque hanging on a wall that grabbed my attention. It had been presented to Lad."

After Terry found the courage, he called.

"Hey Laddie. This is Terry. I don't know what to say."

"Well, how about hello?" said Lad.

§

On June 1, 2002, Lad's first grandchild, Lucas Conrad Troup, was born. And on June, 24, 2004, Rylan Elaine Troup, his second grandchild, came into the world.

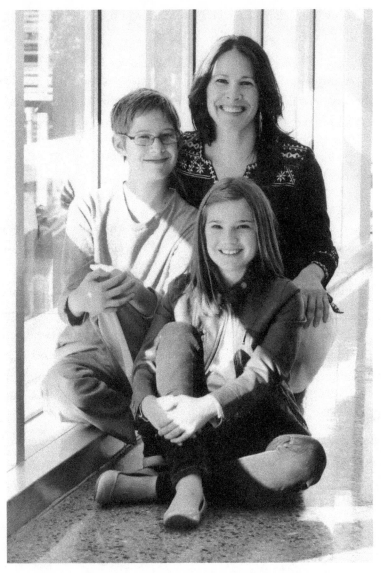

Katie Doctor with children, Lucas and Rylan Troup.
Compliments of Laird Doctor

Chapter 21

What Can I Do?

"What can I do?" asks Lad.

Lad's mind can't shut off. His experience and knowledge in so many areas needs to be tapped into. He can't pick up the phone nor does he have the ability to type on a keyboard. Lad focuses on things he can do.

With Dragon software, Lad stays up-to-date and in contact with others.

He operates his computer, saves and opens files, manages business transactions, stays in contact with friends and family, and continues to explore information that will allow him to think beyond his chair by the sound of his voice.

"Wake up
Go to address line
Type in Mayfield Road
Move down two spaces
Click there
Don't do that
Page down
Copy that
Open file
Paste that
Go to sleep."

§

Years later, Lad immersed himself in the Word and with others who did the same. As his knowledge and understanding grew, Lad is confident that the extreme strength of the "White" was the presence of God.

"I truly believe that I was in the presence of God," said Lad. "The powerful white room or cloud that others have experienced is the presence of God. It is his presence with you. It wasn't a dream. It was real." Throughout the Old Testament, whenever GOD was present it is noted by the descending of a white cloud. Exodus 40:34-35 KJV:

> *Then a cloud covered the tent of the congregation, and the glory of the LORD filled the tabernacle. And Moses was not able to enter into the tent of the congregation, because the cloud abode thereon, and the glory of the LORD filled the tabernacle.*

On more than one occasion, the *North Texas Aero Modelers Club* asked Lad to be their guest speaker to discuss flying one of the many aircraft he had mastered. Club members Danny Volgamore, Gary Saba and John Larsen asked Lad if he would be interested in flying a Radio Controlled Aircraft (RCA).

For most quadriplegics, this question might seem silly and possibly insulting—it takes two hands working simultaneously to fly an RC plane. Lad used his mouth for everything. But Danny, Gary and John probably sensed Lad's passion to do more than what others may think a quadriplegic is capable, especially this quadriplegic.

Lad knew that if he was going to convince other handicapped individuals to think beyond their limitations, he had to be able to prove it. And he needed to convince those who are not handicapped what quadriplegics can successfully accomplish.

Danny, Gary and John thought there was a way for Lad to fly, however, they probably thought it would be more of a fun get-together with many accidents rather than serious flying. They were about to experience what it meant to be Lad Doctor. Mediocre was never a word Lad had learned to spell.

Back at home, Lad immediately put his mind to work to figure out how he could achieve this new goal of flying again, and he shared them with the guys. Lad must ask for help, which has led to more opportunities and friendships. And he wants those who need help to dismiss their pride and just ask.

Danny told Lad that the Lord had given Lad many talents, and together they could successfully complete this possibly *first-time-ever* project. Within a few days, and not without several modifications, Lad had a transmitter attached to his chair and was practicing with the help of a simulator program on his computer.

"A lot of hits and misses along the way to achieve a workable control box," said Lad.

But to fly an RC plane requires the coordination of *two* hands. Lad needed to be able to maintain control of the aircraft while increasing power. He could operate the plane with his mouth, but to be able to do two functions at once should have been the deal-breaker. Instead of Lad focusing on what he could not do, though, he asked himself, "What can I do?"

He remembered that some World War II aircraft had a Blip Switch instead of a throttle. He called Bill and Mike's Hobby Shop and explained his idea. Lad needed them to replicate the Blip Switch for his chair, and the shop did the rest.

Lad now had what the guys would call a *Bump Switch*. With the Bump Switch he could achieve two functions simultaneously: He now had the ability to add 50% power by holding the switch down with his chin for basic aerobatics, and he used his mouth to control the aircraft.

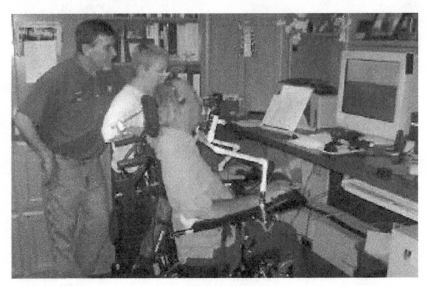

Pre-flight training.
Compliments of Laird Doctor

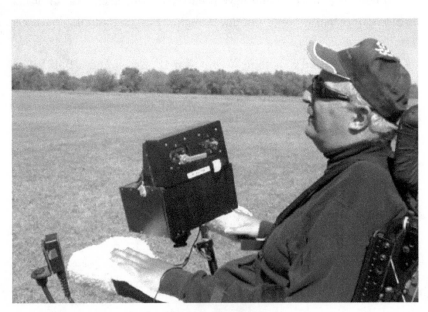

Lad and his incredible modifications.
Compliments of Laird Doctor

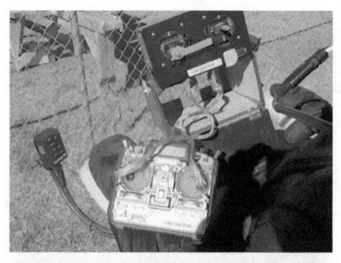

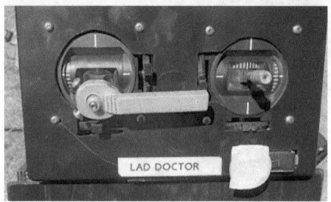

Lad's modified transmitter.
Compliments of Laird Doctor

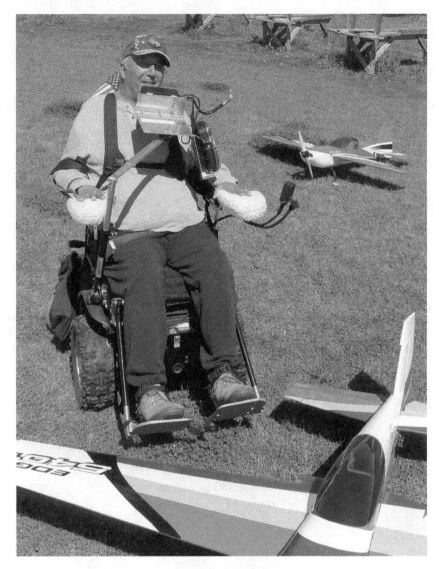

What can I do? *Compliments of Laird Doctor*

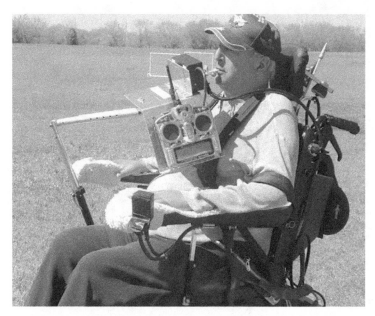

"Think outside the box," says Lad.
Compliments of Laird Doctor

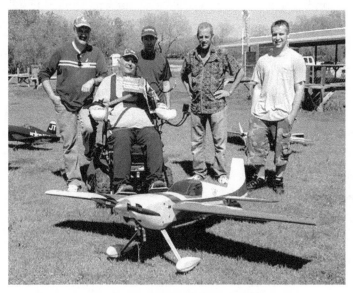

The pilot and his support team.
Compliments of Laird Doctor

There will be life's hardships that can't be adjusted for. If his blood pressure drops too low, it affects his eyesight, which makes it hard to fly a plane.

Before Lad's friend Milo relocated out of state, he made sure Lad's radio-controlled models were in good working order, connecting the wires, loading and unloading them into the trailer and starting the planes. He did everything needed to get the planes ready to fly.

"When I started working with Lad," remembered Milo. "He already had five planes or so. I first started helping Lad put together his big aerobatic 100cc plane called an Extra 300L, I believe. It was a huge project that Lad and I worked on as a team. Lad made all the decisions, and when he needed advice, he asked me since I had a lot of building experience with the big aerobatic gasoline powered planes. Lad excelled in saying stuff like, 'How about if we try this?' At first, I was hesitant because Lad had ideas I had never seen before. Eventually, I learned to trust Lad's new ideas. Sometimes they worked and sometimes they didn't, and we moved on to another idea and didn't cry over spilled milk. Not for a second. Lad was always excellent about accepting a few 'burned meals as part of learning how to cook,' which was one of the many, many, wonderful things I learned from Lad.

"He loves warbirds, naturally. And when building an RC plane, you can spend as much or as little time and money on the details as you wish. Lad's memory of the real planes from front to back was exceptional. This proved very helpful when we added scale details to his yellow Stearman biplane. The fun part was that Lad got resourceful at finding things around the shop to use to make the details. On the Stearman, under the top wing is a gas gauge which I believe we made from a tiny medical syringe because you can't just go to the hobby store and buy one off the shelf the correct size and shape. I think this was a big part of the fun we had building models."

"You want to fly an airplane?" Lad asked. "Well, you can't fly a real airplane. Can't do that. Can you fly a model airplane? You can. It's frustrating. I landed the real plane much better."

The P-38 is one of the few airplanes Lad never had an opportunity to fly, until now. He should have his P-38 up in the air soon.

"I think the Lord wants me to inspire others to think outside the box," said Lad.

"So that's what I am trying to do."

The Dallas Morning News, Monday, August 3, 2009
"Pilot Just Won't Let Injury Keep Him Down"

On a sunny Saturday morning at North Lakes Park in Denton, Laird "Lad" Doctor is hoping the wind slows down a bit. He wants to fly his radio-controlled plane without any problems.

Doctor's friends Danny Volgamore and Gary Saba of the North Texas Aero Modelers Club help him get ready. Saba sets the plane on the runway and adjusts Doctor's wheelchair to ensure that his transmitter is at eye level. Volgamore holds a trainer transmitter—also called a buddy box—connected to Doctor's transmitter to help his friend's plane take flight.

Minutes later, Doctor's red and white plane takes off. With its 78-inch wingspan, the plane flies beautifully—moving slowly like a bird taking its time. While Doctor moves the transmitter with his mouth to maneuver the plane, Saba rotates Doctor's wheelchair, allowing his friend to see the plane during takeoff and landing.

"He is flying," Volgamore said happily. "He is doing it all by himself."

After 20 minutes of flying, Doctor brings his plane back to the runway. The landing is rough, and Doctor appears disappointed. He is hard on himself and wishes he had made a smoother landing.

"The first one was a bit bouncy, that one was a little rough," Saba said

about the second flight of the day. "The gears were pushed down; it's nothing I can't repair...but he is doing better."

For the past 2 ½ years, Doctor, 66, has been learning to fly a radio-controlled plane to continue indulging his passion—being in the sky...

...only by mouth can I move the items and control the parts," he said.[34]

"Every now and then I will flip through an aviation magazine and think, 'Oh! I flew one of those,'" Lad said.

Before moving out of state, Milo helped Lad with daily responsibilities: paying the bills, fishing limbs from the roof, customizing Lad's RC planes, and being a friend.

"He is irreplaceable," said Lad.

§

Lad's hope is for others to look beyond their chair and live life.

"Just to be out in nature is to be in the Cathedral of God," Lad reflected. "Look at the complexity of all living things that he has given us. The veins in a leaf. He has certainly shown us only a sliver of his loving kindness and all for his glory. Life doesn't end with the physical circumstances in which you may find yourself. It won't be easy. I truly believe with a deep and committed faith in God. Your life, regardless of condition, is going to be richer *with him*. I pray for the riches of life to be yours, but ultimately, the choice is yours.

"Turn off the television and start thinking outside the box. Reach out to those who can help your dreams come true. I have made some wonderful new friends. *With God's help*, join me in finding a way to accomplish a better life."

§

Lad had acquired an impressive assortment of over thirty guns that he used in competitive sports, such as trap, skeet, sporting clays, and Helice ZZ target shooting. Lad owned a nice collection, which would not come as a shock to fellow members of the *Dallas Gun Club*, or to those who knew him as a young boy. But he never had the opportunity to fire some of them, and because of his inability to control his environment, repairmen and medical staff stole many of them.

"Anything that could be picked up and carried out I've lost," said Lad. "Including my favorite pair of Lucchese boots and watch. And because of this, anything of value left has been removed from my home."

His greatest treasures are now being put away in heaven!

§

"Wow! Unbelievable!" said Jim. "How?"

Lad cannot hold his head straight up or down. It will always be tilted a little to the left. And yet, with all these obstacles, he hit the mark.

"If I can fly a plane, then I can shoot a gun!" Lad told himself. "What can I do? How can I shoot a gun?"

Lad called the Department of Public Safety.

"I'm a quadriplegic. Can I obtain a concealed handgun license?"

"You can't aim the gun," said the representative.

"I can," said Lad.

"You can't use a laser," the rep challenged.

"Don't need one," replied Lad.

"How do you intend to aim the gun?" he asked.

"Can I obtain a gun license?" Lad asked.

"If you can find a way to pass the test," he replied.

That was all Lad needed to know. He immediately contacted an old pilot buddy and asked if he would be willing to put his ideas on paper and build the mockup. With safety a priority, they used a Glock.

Together, Lad and his friend, who owned a large machining company, completed the blueprint, built prototypes and, when they finally got it right, sent the mockup to a mechanic friend. In a short time, Lad's idea was successfully mounted to his chair.

One evening, shortly before weekly Bible study group began, Lad asked Jim Coffee if he would administer the tests required to issue him a concealed handgun license. Jim, the Captain of the University of North Texas Police Department, agreed to put Lad to the test. Jim was also a concealed handgun instructor and maintained the authority to issue the license.

On the day of the test, Lad puffed and sipped his 400 pound wheelchair out of the van and onto the gun range.

"Do you need help?" Jim asked.

"Nope," said Lad.

"You can't use a laser," Jim told him.

Lad lined up his chair 21 feet from the target. *Pop pop pop pop pop!* The sound lingered in the air.

"Wow! Unbelievable!" said Jim. Lad had hit the target just right of the bullseye.

"I could have done a little better with a little adjustment," Lad said, "but this works."

"How?" Jim asked, dumbfounded.

"Look beside my right knee."

Concealed in a black bag strapped to the side of Lad's chair was the gun. Without a laser, Lad had hit the target.

"With the assistance of a camera," explained Lad. "I adjust my wheelchair until I have my sites on the target. Then I push the switch with my mouth to fire. The semi-automatic gun allows me several shots before needing to be reloaded."

Jim, still a little shell-shocked, said, "Line it up and shoot again."

Pop pop pop pop pop!

Again, Lad hit inside the target rings.

Jim stood there with his hand over his mouth. "I don't believe it. I just don't believe it. You have just got to come show this to my officers. You shoot better than they do."

Lad received his license.

The little boy who had once pressed his nose on the glass of the gun case hoping to hold one in his hands didn't know at the time that he didn't need to hold one in his hands to hit the target.

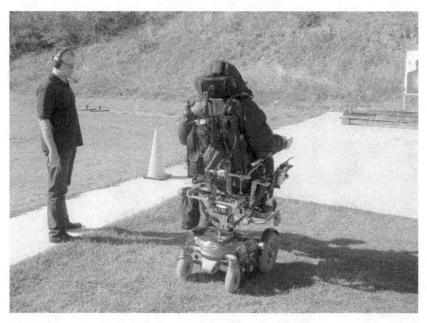

Aiming his gun. *Compliments of Laird Doctor*

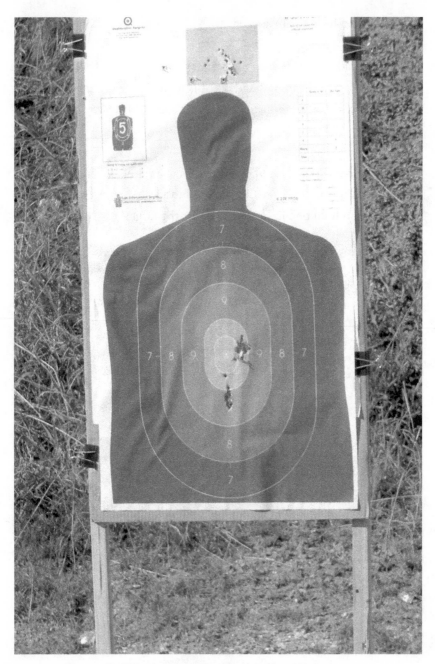

Lad hits the target. *Compliments of Laird Doctor*

Chapter 22

Hang in There, Lad!

Lad's cardiologist walked in with a student who said, "The doctor told me all about you, your great disposition, good attitude and accomplishments."

"Lad is very unusual," the cardiologist added. "The life expectancy of someone in Lad's condition is between five and seven years."

"I'm on borrowed time," said Lad.

§

Lad is writing a book entitled, From Where I Sit. In it, he will detail the ignored and overlooked needs of a quadriplegic by the medical profession. Lad is showing the world what can happen when anyone in his condition is not placed by a wall next to the nurse's station, out of the way. Lad is on God's schedule, not a statistical chart.

"I have always warned that if I catch a cold, I'll be in intensive care," he reflected. "Well, a nurse had been exposed to the flu, and thinking that she was well enough, she came to work."

On Saturday, February 4, 2017, within hours after the infected nurse arrived at work, Lad was in the emergency room suffering from a fairly violent case of influenza, on death's door.

On Monday, February 6, 2017, there was no sign of improvement. Lad was sedated and put through aggressive treatments for several hours. If he did not improve by the next day, there would be little hope for his survival. Unbeknownst to any of the medical staff, many prayers were being said for Lad's recovery.

On Wednesday, February 8, 2017, Lad was able to return home and could take some of his medication by mouth and started eating again. It was a very tumultuous ordeal.

On Thursday, February 9, 2017, Lad experienced complications and was transported back to the emergency room by ambulance. He was able to return home, but never got out of bed and was on oxygen 24 hours a day. Nursing staff focused on his respiratory care and nutrition.

Lad has been a miracle over and over and over.

"I have mentioned to a lot of people," said Lad, "that this year has been an interesting one for overcoming some physical problems. And that all miracles were with the help of the Lord. I was so far gone. They just kept pounding on me, pumping things into me, yelling at me."

It's a miracle that Lad is alive today. It hit him fast.

"The protocol is if I need any respiratory work, to call Michael Jouett immediately."

Michael dropped everything and rushed to the hospital to start working on Lad. But the hospital staff stopped him due to legal concerns and fears. Michael Jouett had to first propose a persuasive argument to the medical staff. The hospital staff wanted no part of allowing Michael to touch Lad, let alone work on him, even though he was the one person who had been through it all with him and knew what worked and what didn't.

"Finally, he must have been allowed to work on me," said Lad. "Because, as I understand it, after the hospital staff failed to get any air into me, Michael was then allowed to try his manipulations, but they weren't working either. My lungs were filling faster than Michael could clean them out. The hospital had no other choice but to run tubes into my lungs. My temperature was high and, in the midst of everything else going wrong, my heart had them concerned enough to call my cardiologist."

"Given Lad's heart history," said the cardiologist. "It will either kill him or it won't, but there is nothing we can do about it."

"They could not do heart surgery on me in my condition," said Lad. "I can remember Suzi and Michael saying, 'Stay with us Lad. Stay with us Lad. Stay with us. It's Michael. It's Michael. Suzi's here. Stay with us.'"

At that time, prayers ascended for Lad from all across Fort Worth and Dallas. Lad remembered trying to reach out to Michael and Suzi as they frantically worked to revive him.

"Stay with us Lad!" yelled Suzi.

"I can remember trying to get Michael's attention. In the midst of all the chaos, all of a sudden, I had the most glorious feeling of relief and peace. I tried to tell Michael, 'I'm at peace. I am at Peace.' I think that I must have been ready to die. I don't know why the Lord presented that to me at that moment. The feeling was real and it was significant. I felt it mentally as well as physically. I tried to tell Michael, twice. Man, it was something. That peace, boy it felt so good."

As Lad held on, his good friend, Greg Storm, walked into his hospital room. But not before the medical staff covered him from head to foot in special garments, including a mask, full-length apron and gloves.

"They wanted no part of my germs in that room," said Greg.

Equipment, tubes, monitors, and the ominous beeping sounds they emitted echoed around the room.

"Funny thing was," said Greg. "I had never seen Lad in anything other than his wheelchair. Strange the things that take getting used to, things your brain struggles with."

Lad still wasn't responding. The nurse briefed Greg on the immediate plan of action, which was to reduce his medication in hopes of getting a response. If it didn't work, then when Katie arrived, they would remove his breathing tube.

The medical staff asked Greg if he would try to get Lad to respond. Greg was an emotional wreck. His friend needed to be back in his wheelchair.

"Lad, let's go grab some beer and get out of here!" said Greg.

Immediately Lad responded.

It was a miracle indeed. The doctor put Lad back under until Katie arrived.

"He certainly 'responded' as though he recognized me," said Greg. "And raised his eyebrows. Everyone in the room (me, the nurse, Lad's attendant, and the doctor) all agreed that he 'perked up.'"

"The flu caused inflammation in the airways of his lungs, producing a lot of thin secretions," explained Michael Jouett. "This resulted in his needing to be helped with coughing almost continuously. He became exhausted and, since he is partly ventilator-dependent, we decided to take him to the hospital for his safety. This was a decision we would eventually regret. While in the hospital, they unnecessarily gave him some very strong antibiotics which caused, we believe, a very severe delirium. Development of delirium in the hospital is considered a grave prognostic sign. After a few days, they moved him out of the ICU to a regular patient room, where, apparently, they expected him to die. At that point, we and his daughter insisted to take him home, and his regular pulmonary doctor agreed to discontinue all antibiotics. At home, we sent respiratory therapists to treat him four times a day for ten days to clear his lungs and to wean him from oxygen. Within a few days, the delirium began to subside, and within seven to ten days his mentation had returned to normal. Within four to six weeks he was able to fully resume his regular daily activities."

Sometime later, Lad's psychologist rolled his wheelchair next to Lad's and said, "Just think, that peace you felt is just a foretaste of what heaven will be like."

Lad's purpose has not yet been fulfilled. After this episode Lad feels that he can't plan for any tomorrows.

"They were trying to get my heart in order while trying to get me breathing," said Lad. "It was an eye-opening experience."

Sometime later, Greg Storm and Lad discussed a rash of military accidents. "These guys aren't getting any flying time," said Lad. "I don't care what you do in a simulator, it ain't the same."

Lad, was back.

§

Hi Stella, thanks for sending the email. I had an opportunity to watch the video and to speak to my friend Rick Veit who was with me when this happened. I recall that we were amongst thousands anticipating the launch of the flight of Naval Warbird flight. We were shocked when we saw a Corsair somersault before landing up-side down and catch fire. As the seconds ticked by waiting for the fire equipment to arrive, we felt helpless to do anything so we just locked arms and began to pray. We had no idea who we were praying for but we knew he needed prayer. After that we just left and went back to our hotel. We figured there would be no more flying for the day but we also were so emotionally drained having witnessed such a horrible scene.

I was so glad to hear that Laird had survived and I sent an email to try to encourage him at a low point in his life. I cannot imagine waking up the next day totally crippled and in pain.

I want you to know that this next part I share from my heart. I know that having never walked in Lairds shoes I cannot understand his situation. I do believe in Jesus as my deliverer and my hope of eternal life in heaven. I do not believe that God orchestrates things like this but I do believe he knows and he cares. I do believe that he can use all of us each day of our lives to glorify him. I have looked online and it appears Laird has used his life to help others and for this I respect him greatly. I also am glad to hear of our mutual hope of heaven. Our current life is temporary, but I believe that one day we will all wake up in a home that is beyond our ability to comprehend. We will awake with perfect bodies and perfect minds. No physical or mental pain and just pure joy. That is my hope of heaven and I pray that Laird would continue to live each day serving God with his life and with that amazing hope of an eternal life beyond description.

Blessings to you both!
Rick Millham

PS Semper Fidelis is Latin for Forever Faithful.

Chapter 23

Cavanaugh's

Greg and I could not wait! Lad had promised to give us a personal tour of Cavanaugh Flight Museum and we were counting the days.

Lad amazed us even before he entered the museum's front door. The wheelchair ramp was extremely narrow, extremely short and at a perfect 90-degree angle. If I had grabbed his wheelchair, the wheels would have slipped off the edge of the slender strip of pavement. With puffs and sips, he made that sharp turn with both wheels teetering at the edge of both sides of the sidewalk. Amazing! Simply amazing!

When he entered the museum, he came alive. He was home. His energy and knowledge was magnetic. A patron shuffled closer, hoping to catch every word. Lad explained the how, what and why of every aspect of every plane. He knew the history behind every drop of paint used on a plane. A spot of rust or a flat tire stirred his emotion. We studied each plane as he brought it back to life.

"...I sat jump seat in the B-29 a few times," Lad said. "You lumbered down the runway forever, you kind of pick up the landing gear. Doesn't climb worth a shit. It stays low to the ground a long time. ...The Connie was designed by Howard Hughes."

As Lad graciously led us through Cavanaugh Flight Museum, he transformed the place from a museum to a place where excitement and life once transpired. A place where celebrations, laughter, honors, surprise, handshakes, and friendships were made.

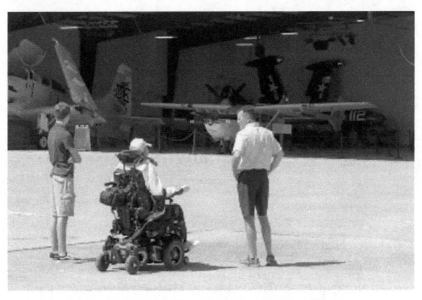

Lucas, Lad and Greg Storm at Cavenaugh Flight Museum.
Compliments of Greg Storm

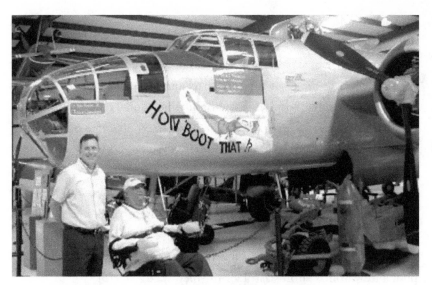

Greg Storm and Lad at Cavenaugh Flight Museum.
Compliments of Greg Storm

"Being a quadriplegic doesn't mean that you give up on life," said Lad. "Those with my level of injury generally live out their lives in a nursing home and fed heavy doses of valium while staring at a television. I just can't be satisfied with that. It's not the way I lived and it's not the way I will die when the Lord calls me. The accident is just another blessing in disguise.

"I thought that I could do anything and everything. I did not need God. I never even thought about him. I just went on my merry way. Now I can see that all of those things were by the Grace of God. Opportunities I thought I was choosing to do weren't really my doing. I know that now. He's got my attention. I can't do anything else except what he wants me to do. And that is, to use my mind and my experiences to think outside the box, achieve and inspire others to do the same."

God does exist and Jesus died on the cross to wash away our sins. Lad experienced the presence of God, the love of Jesus and the road to heaven. His story is real. The devil could not allow Lad's powerful message

219

to reach the lost. The devil threw huge roadblocks—depression, fear, a difficult trial, divorce, and being seconds from death.

Through the grace of God, Lad was not burned; Eric Johnston was at the right place at the right time. Michael and Suzi Jouett walked into his life. Greg was at the hospital at the right time. God's peace and strength and a victory over illness that can't be explained all came about at the right time.

Through prayer, there was no way the devil would overcome.

In Addison, Texas, at Cavanaugh Flight Museum, the WWII war birds remain frozen in time. But if you're really fortunate, as you stroll past a powerful plane that once carried brave men safely through war, maybe you will have the joy of meeting that passionate and experienced pilot and warbirds enthusiast, Laird Ashley "Lad" Doctor.

Today, the Lord lives in Lad's heart as his Lord and Master.

He's got my attention.

"It was white. It wasn't a dream or a hallucination. It was real. The strength of the intense "white" was very significant," said Lad.

§

Acts 2: 17-21. In the last days, God says,
I will pour out my Spirit on all people. Your sons and daughters will prophesy, your young men will see visions, your old men will dream dreams.

§

Laird Ashley "Lad" Doctor. Naval Pilot, Vietnam Veteran and Witness. Lad, Thank you for your service, then and now.

Appendix

Some of aircraft Lad had flown:

The Pitts Special
Christian Eagle II
Piper J-3 Cub
PT-17 Stearman Kaydet
Messerschmitt Me 109/Hispano HA-1112
Grumman TBM Avenger
Grumman FM-2 Wildcat
Vultee BT-13 Valiant
North American AT-6/SNJ Texan
Supermarine Spitfire Mk. VIII
Douglas AD-5 Skyraider
North American T-28 Trojan
Mig-15/17

Grumman S2F-1 Tracker

North American/Canadair F-86 Sabre

Grumman F9F-2B Panther

Cessna 0-2A Skymaster

Douglas A-26C Invader

North American B-25J Mitchell

Ryan PT-22 Recruit

Piper L-4J

Fairchild PT-19 Cornell

Republic P-47N Thunderbolt

T-2A Buckeye

RA5C Vigilante

L-29 Delfin

F4U-4 Corsair

T-34 Mentor

AF-8 Cougar

TF-9 Cougar

References

1   Ebert, Karl, Collar, Jim, and Hummel, Alex. "Bearcat, Corsair Collide at EAA During Takeoff". Oshkosh Daily Northwestern, 30 July 1999.

2   "1939 Boston Red Sox Roster". *Baseball Reference*. n.d. 18 July 2020. https://www.baseball-reference.com/teams/BOS/1939-roster.shtml.

3   Bergin, Bob. "Charlie Bond's Air Duels". *Warfare History Network*. n.d. 18 July 2020. https://warfarehistorynetwork.com/2015/11/18/charlie-bonds-air-duels/.

4   Tibbets, Paul W., with Stebbins, Clair and Franken, Harry. The Tibbets Story. Briarcliff Manor, New York: Stein and Day, Inc., 1978. 161, 168.

5   Vukovich, Bill Jr. "Page 5 Vukovich Family Biography by Bones Bourcier." *The Vukovich Racing Legacy*. 22 November 2012. 18 July 2020. http://www.billvukovich.com/?attachment_id=1806.

6   "Invention Awards to Ames Employees." *The Astrogram, Volume XIV, Number 6.* 6 January 1972. 18 July 2020. https://history.arc.nasa.gov/Astrogram/astrogram_1972_1.pdf

7   Carlson, Peter. "Nikita Khrushchev Goes to Hollywood". *Smithsonian Magazine.* July 2009. 18 July 2020. https://www.smithsonianmag.com/history/nikita-khrushchev-goes-to-hollywood-30668979/?sessionguid=3720c493-2ea9-a752-1aa9-062e83999a57&noist=&page=4

8   Ibid.

9   Castagnera, Dr. Jim, Esq., Chief Consultant, Holland Media Services. "The History Place™ presents The Vietnam War: America Commits 1961-1964". *The History Place.* n.d. 18 July 2020. http://www.historyplace.com/unitedstates/vietnam/index-1961.html

10 Ibid.

11 Ibid.

12 "Shelter Supplies Due within Ninety Days". *Valley State Daily Sundial,* 26 March 1963.

13 "Students Puff, Then Huff as VSC Smoking Study Begins." *Valley State Daily Sundial,* 3 November 1966, p. 12.

14 Leung, Lily. "Vietnam Vets Blame Jet Guns for Their Hepatitis C". *The Orange County Register.* 17 February 2016. 18 July 2020. https://www.ocregister.com/2016/02/17/vietnam-vets-blame-jet-guns-for-their-hepatitis-c/

15 "Optical landing system". *Wikipedia, the free encyclopedia.* n.d. 18 July 2020. https://en.wikipedia.org/wiki/Optical_landing_system

16 Johnston, Erik. "Veteran Tales Interview #3 'Lad' Doctor". *YouTube, ErikJohnston.* 19 January 2011. 18 July 2020. https://www.youtube.com/user/ErikJohnston/search?query=lad+doctor

17 Ibid.

18 Ibid.

19 Ibid.

20 Nolte, John. "Jane Fonda on 'Hanoi Jane' Scandal: 'It's Horrible for me to Think of that.'" *Breitbart*. 26 July 2018. 18 July 2020. https://www.breitbart.com/entertainment/2018/07/26/jane-fonda-on-hanoi-jane-scandal-its-horrible-for-me-to-think-of-that/

21 "Air Force Plant 42." *dreamlandresort.com*. n.d. 18 July 2020. https://www.dreamlandresort.com/black_projects/plant42.htm

22 Moeser, Sharon. "Career Day at Plant 42 Takes Off." *Los Angeles Times*, 30 April 1994.

23 Turner, Betty Stagg. *Out of the Blue and Into History*. Lake Forest, Illinois: Aviatrix Publishing Inc, 2001.

24 Tibbets, Paul W., with Stebbins, Clair and Franken, Harry. *The Tibbets Story*. Briarcliff Manor, New York: Stein and Day, Inc., 1978. 168.

25 "Ace in a Day – Oct 12, 1944". *Chuckyeager.org*. n.d. 18 July 2020. http://www.chuckyeager.org/ace-in-a-day/#

26 "Chance Vought F4U Corsair XF4U-1: Genesis". *f4ucorsair.com*. n.d. 18 July 2020. http://f4ucorsair.com/history.html

27 Ebert, Karl, Collar, Jim, and Hummel, Alex. "Bearcat, Corsair Collide at EAA During Takeoff". *Oshkosh Daily Northwestern*, 30 July 1999.

28 Ibid.

29 "Pilot Seriously Hurt as Planes Collide at EAA Fly-in". *The Capital Times*. 30 July 1999.

30 Ebert, Karl, Collar, Jim, and Hummel, Alex. "Texas Man Hospitalized in Critical Condition". *Oshkosh Daily Northwestern*, 30 July 1999, p 1.

31 Ibid.

32 Ibid.

33 *Laird DOCTOR and Linda Doctor, Appellants, v. Howard E. PARDUE and Experimental Aircraft Association, Inc., Appellees*. September 15, 2005 Court of Appeals of Texas, Houston (1st Dist.).

34 "Pilot Just Won't Let Injury Keep Him Down." *The Dallas Morning News*. 3 August 2009.

About the Author

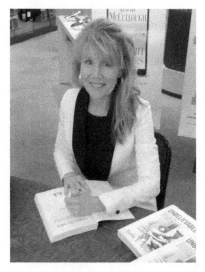

Photo courtesy of Ben Merritt

Stella Brooks is the author of *Unbelievable: The Unmasking of Dr. Harrison Miller Moseley,* the true story of a small boy who defeats huge physical and psychological challenges to become a brilliant scientist working among the Who's Who on the Atomic Bomb. The enormous research coupled with Brooks' style brings the reader into the scene creating a cinematic wonder.

With that same cinematic flair, *Grounded* will forever change lives and empower those the world forgot.

CPSIA information can be obtained
at www.ICGtesting.com
Printed in the USA
LVHW090745161020
668887LV00008B/426